CHANGING THE CULTURE OF
ACADEMIC MEDICINE

CHANGING THE CULTURE OF
Academic Medicine

{ *Perspectives of Women Faculty* }

Linda H. Pololi

Dartmouth College Press
Hanover, New Hampshire

PUBLISHED BY
UNIVERSITY PRESS OF NEW ENGLAND
HANOVER AND LONDON

Dartmouth College Press
Published by University Press of New England
One Court Street, Lebanon NH 03766
www.upne.com
© 2010 Trustees of Dartmouth College
Manufactured in the United States of America
Designed by Katherine B. Kimball
Typeset in Sabon by Integrated Publishing Solutions

University Press of New England is a member
of the Green Press Initiative. The paper used in this book
meets their minimum requirement for recycled paper.

For permission to reproduce any of the material in this
book, contact Permissions, University Press of New
England, One Court Street, Lebanon NH 03766; or visit
www.upne.com

Library of Congress Cataloging-in-Publication Data
Pololi, Linda H.
Changing the culture of academic medicine : perspectives
of women faculty / Linda H. Pololi.
   p. ; cm.
Includes bibliographical references and index.
ISBN 978-1-58465-567-1 (pbk. : alk. paper)
   1. Women in medicine.   2. Women college teachers.
3. Medical colleges—Faculty.   I. Title.
   [DNLM: 1. Faculty, Medical.   2. Physicians, Women—
psychology.   3. Academic Medical Centers—organization
& administration.   4. Organizational Culture.   5. Prejudice.   6. Sex Factors. W 18 P778c 2010]
   R692.P65 2010
   610.82—dc22   2010013166

5 4 3 2 1

*For my husband, Athanasius Anagnostou,
fellow traveler who took time with love
and generosity to be with me in academic
medicine.*

*For my loving parents, Eva Berger and
Francesco Pololi, who always supported
my choices.*

*For my children, Anthony Anagnostou and
Alistair Reader, who are my finest
teachers.*

Injustice anywhere is injustice everywhere.
—Martin Luther King Jr.

CONTENTS

ACKNOWLEDGMENTS

A great many talented men and women who care deeply about relationships and connection in medicine made this work possible. As I reflect on the individuals I want to thank for their collaboration and encouragement of my work and of this book, I realize that the hallmark of these people is their generosity of spirit, their acceptance of my (and others') perspectives and differences, and the welcome and consistent support they have provided me, professionally and personally. They demonstrate the amalgam of "heartset" and mindset for me.

It has been a privilege and rewarding journey to carry out this work with my collaborators and school partners. They all demonstrated extraordinary courage and commitment to investigate highly sensitive professional areas in the hope of improving the lives of faculty, students, and patients alike. I thank the deans of the initial five C - Change schools, Deborah Powell, Jim Scott, Sandy Williams, Paul Roth, and Michael Rosenblatt, for embarking on the C - Change project with vision, open-mindedness, and willingness to explore for the good of their faculty and institutions. I am exceptionally appreciative of all the faculty who participated in the interviews for the research projects. We listened to their aspirations and stories with great admiration. Phyllis Carr, Sharon Knight, and Peter Conrad collaborated in the C - Change second set of interviews. I am very grateful for their talented contributions to that portion of the research study. An early grant for the initial interview study from Kathleen Christensen of the Alfred P. Sloan Foundation launched a new phase in my career.

The Josiah Macy, Jr. Foundation funded the National Initiative on Gender, Culture and Leadership in Medicine, C - Change, with extraordinary generosity. June Osborn, the then-president of the Macy Foundation, was an inspiring champion for the Initiative together with Marc Nivet, the Foundation's COO. The continuing support of her Board members and her successor George Thibault allowed the work of C - Change to proceed. Wanda Jones and Anna Kindermann at the U.S. DHHS Office on Women's Health contributed support, both moral and instrumental, to the study and pulled together a collaborative funding agreement among five federal agencies to provide us with supplemental resources. I also thank the late Ruth Kirschstein at NIH for her early encouragement, Vivian Pinn in the Office of Research on Women's Health at NIH for her support together with Sabrina Matoff-Stepp at the Health Resources and Services Administration, Shakeh Kaftarian at the Agency for Health Care Research and Quality, Yvonne Green at the Centers for Disease Control and Prevention, and Betty Lee Hawks at the Office on Minority Health.

In my career at four medical schools and Brandeis University, many colleagues stand out for their friendship, advice, and support. I am especially indebted to Marsha Fretwell, Carol Tresolini, David Giansiracusa, Connie Cardasis, Loring Conant, Jordan Cohen, William Salazar, Jo Solet, and Hilda and Merton Kahne—each a kind and wise colleague with a strong moral compass. They were instrumental in helping me clarify the focus of my work, and they embody the very best aspects of academic leaders. Arlene Ash, David Kern, Ed Krupat, Michael Goldstein, Lisa Cooper, and Geno Schnell have been truly outstanding colleagues in the C - Change project. They are intellectual powerhouses and thinking partners, kindred spirits, and personal friends. I thank colleagues from my time at East Carolina University—Diana Antonnacci, Jack Rose, David Weismiller, Lorrie Basnight, and Julius Mallette—and all the fine faculty members who participated in my faculty development and mentoring programs there. I have fond memories of those days. Colleagues and concepts from the American Academy on Physician and Patient (recently renamed the American Academy on Communication in Healthcare) were very influential in my work. Mack Lipkin has been a trustworthy mentor to me for over two decades and Doug Dickson more recently. Thanks also to Penny Williamson, Rich Frankel, and Charlie O'Leary for their guidance on facilitation. I am deeply grateful to Parker Palmer, Marcy Jackson, and colleagues I met at their facilitator preparation courses who helped me integrate the concepts of their Center for Courage and Renewal into my work. I thank Rosalind Chait Barnett, Lotte Bailyn, and Millie Solomon for their encouragement of the research studies described here, and Lynn Goldsmith, Richard Alfred, and Sallie Carlisle for their unstinting friendship during difficult times. Stephanie Golden assisted greatly in organizing the material for my manuscript and making it more accessible to a wider readership through her many helpful questions, and Janet Paraschos was generous in her help with additional editing. Phyllis Deutsch has been a remarkably patient and supportive publishing editor.

The truth is that this book and its described research effort would not have happened without the welcoming and nurturing environment of the Women's Studies Research Center (WSRC) at Brandeis University. I am inspired by the intellectual curiosity and openness exhibited by my fellow scholars there. The interdisciplinary nature of the Center is exhilarating, and I have been fascinated by the helpful perspectives on my work of economists, psychologists, sociologists, lawyers, politicians, writers, historians, artists, and musicians. Similarly, I continue to find great pleasure in learning of my Brandeis colleagues' own different disciplines and research studies. The abundance of diverse intellectual riches found in this unusual scholarly community models the culture of academic cross-fertilization, partnership, and companionship I tried so hard over the years to bring to my students and faculty in medical schools. I particularly thank my fellow scholars in the WSRC Social Issues Research Group for their plentiful and consistently helpful feedback and subversive insights—with humor and deep scholarship—on my research and this book.

Most of all, I am grateful to Shula Reinharz, founding director of the Women's Studies Research Center at Brandeis. Shula is a visionary and inspirational leader who created and has maintained in the Center a truly happy environment characterized by intellectual curiosity, creativity, transparency, and inclusiveness. It has been my great good fortune to work with Shula these past years, and I have learned much from her example.

The collegial atmosphere of the WSRC extends to the support offices at Brandeis. Whether it is help in grant writing, budgeting, or scholarly expertise in research methodology, I have always encountered a very generous attitude—"That's a good idea, I'll help!" In particular, I thank Provost Marty Krauss, President Jehuda Reinharz, and Stan Bolotin in Research Administration. I am grateful to Kerri O'Connor who worked painstakingly on the many manuscript revisions and Patricia Plante for her help with C - Change.

Finally, my thanks to my husband Athanasius Anagnostou for his great love and companionship on my journey, and to my two sons, Anthony Anagnostou and Alistair Reader, who exemplify my hopes for the next generation.

CHANGING THE CULTURE OF
ACADEMIC MEDICINE

chapter 1   The Culture of Academic Medicine
through the Lens of Women's Experience

{ Over my career, I've been very moved by the enormous trust that a patient can
place in a physician and the privilege the physician has of holding that trust. It's
like a sacred space. It is a place for trust. I believe that students and physicians
need to understand that this is their privilege, and how unusual that is, and
what an enormous responsibility that is. And also, how rewarding it is as a
physician to be able to enter into that relationship, that intimacy with someone
that would normally take many years to develop—if you ever developed it—with
a friend, or even a partner or family member.
—Senior woman faculty member }

A medical school education and a career in medicine are truly great priv-
ileges in life. The opportunities to explore the human condition so closely
and to assuage human suffering are profound experiences for men and
women both. Yet the institution of academic medicine that enables them
to pursue this calling is in difficulty.

Academic medicine, the pride and keystone of American health care,
is usually based at a medical center that includes a medical school and its
affiliated teaching hospital and clinics. Highly accomplished physicians
and research scientists serve as faculty and deliver on academic medicine's
tripartite mission: medical education, patient care, and biomedical research. Medical students and physicians are trained to serve the nation,
researchers pursue new knowledge or treatments, and a great number
and variety of patients are cared for by some of the best physicians in the
world. The fundamental goal of all these activities is to improve the
health and well-being of the population.

This book argues that academic medicine falls short in its stated mission and responsibilities and explores the reasons for this shortcoming

through the lens of the lives and work experiences of women academic faculty. It describes in these women's words both their passionate devotion to their work and the stubborn problems they encounter at their medical schools. Then it argues that the solution to these problems, and those of academic medicine in general, is actually already present in the form of an increasingly diverse faculty and medical student body—a tremendous reservoir of talent, passion, and dedication that can be mobilized to better address the nation's health care needs. For this to happen, however, the present culture of the academic medical establishment must undergo drastic change.

The work presented here is based on two large series of scientifically structured interviews with women medical faculty. Their stories shine a bright and often unfavorable light on the overall culture of academic medicine. Our interviewees make a strong case that problems they experience in this culture are in fact integral to the larger issues plaguing our health care: a national health system that distributes its services and resources unevenly and thus unjustly; academic medical centers that fail to live up to their stated missions; and patients often dissatisfied with the care they receive or the way doctors communicate with them. From our interviews and my own career in academic medicine, I am well aware that many male medical faculty face similar dilemmas. However, women in academic medicine occupy a quasi-outsider status that gives them a perspective that men by and large do not share.

Although this book does not focus on the vital and informative perspectives of faculty who are members of ethnically or racially underrepresented minority groups, their views are equally important and were also fiercely sought in our interview and national studies. Nor does the book address issues faced by women physicians who practice outside academic medicine or compare women medical faculty with professional women in other academic fields.

The experiences of women medical faculty, though varied, highlight a number of troublesome questions about academic medicine:

1. Why do so many talented women physicians and medical researchers fail to realize their full potential and become leaders? (This is no longer a "pipeline" issue because for decades women have been entering medical schools in large numbers.)

2. Medical school faculty emphasize that they love their work of teaching, clinical practice, and research and find it richly rewarding. In that case, why are there are such high levels of burnout among them? Both women and men are often so discontented that many leave academic medicine and declare that they would not recommend to others that they become physicians.

3. Why is there a startling level of unethical behavior among medical researchers?

4. Why are we seeing an erosion of idealism among medical students, which has implications for their future practice of medicine?

5. Why are medical schools unable to recruit and retain appropriate numbers of faculty members from underrepresented ethnic and racial minority groups?

Much has been written about medical schools from the perspective of students, but little literature exists from the point of view of faculty, particularly women faculty. Yet their views of the institution are extremely valuable for, as we will see, they offer insights unavailable to those positioned solidly in the center of the culture.

How This Book Came About

I write as a former medical faculty member myself and also as a medical educator who created and provided successful faculty development programs for many years, which I found very rewarding. After medical school and internal medicine specialty training at the University of London and a fellowship in hematology and oncology in Chicago, I accepted an academic faculty position at the University of Illinois College of Medicine where I cared for patients in the hospital wards and in outpatient clinics. My federally funded research focused on understanding how blood cells develop from stem cells and the application of this knowledge to bone marrow transplantation. However, as I became more interested in disease prevention and behavioral change than in ordering chemotherapy treatments that only variably prolonged patients' lives and often made them miserable, I took a position as Assistant Professor of Medicine in the Division of General Internal Medicine at Brown University Medical School. At Brown, along with my interests in psychosocial and preventive medicine,

I also developed a passion for medical education (Pololi et al. 1994; Pololi 1995; Pololi and Potter 1996; Pololi et al. 1998b).

Some years later, I became assistant dean at East Carolina University School of Medicine, in rural eastern North Carolina, and worked on innovations in medical student education and on the professional development of faculty (Pololi et al. 2003). I was fascinated by the possibility of creating environments that facilitated learning for both medical students and faculty, improved continuity in care and teaching, and enhanced physician–patient communication (Pololi and Price 2000). For example, we completely restructured a major lecture-based course into a clinically based course taught in small student groups. It has remained largely unchanged for a decade and, I'm told, is still the course medical students enjoy most. This 200-hour "Introduction to Medicine" course was redesigned to be learner-centered, using patient problems that the students had to research. We introduced other innovative ways of learning, such as training people to act as "standardized patients" for the students, and offered students concurrent longitudinal community-based clinical experience with a doctor so that they had an integrated appreciation of the different dimensions of illness: biological, psychological, and social. To further support this learning, we introduced reflective journaling and facilitated "reflection groups" in which students could discuss with peers and faculty their impressions and responses to these early and formative clinical experiences and the meaningfulness and responsibilities of the professional roles they were starting to assume (Pololi et al. 2001b; Pololi and Frankel 2001).

Along the way, I came to feel strongly that the key to successful enhancement of the student educational curriculum had to be a strengthened faculty education process because the faculty themselves knew only traditional teaching methods. For this purpose, I developed and implemented a series of faculty development programs that integrated a focus on relationships and personal awareness to support faculty professional education (Pololi et al. 1998a, 2001a; Pololi and Frankel 2005).

In addition to feeling a deep and sustaining joy from feedback about those programs, I also became very interested in cross-cultural communication in patient care and with faculty, and in distributive justice (Pololi et al. 2000; Putsch and Pololi 2004). I continued in my role as assistant dean and a professor of medicine, and, based on my faculty development work, the Office on Women's Health of the U.S. Department of Health and Human Services selected and funded us as one of four vanguard National Centers of Leadership in Academic Medicine. Our charge was to design and implement model mentoring programs for medical faculty (Pololi et al. 2002, 2004; Pololi and Knight 2005; Pololi 2006). I continue to consult on faculty mentoring programs at a number of organizations and medical schools. I also served briefly as vice-chancellor for education and professor of medicine at a New England medical school, which gave me additional perspectives on the need for culture change.

Having spent so much time with both senior and junior faculty, I came to understand their often expressed feelings of loneliness and isolation; of heavy responsibility and feelings of inadequacy; their aspirations to bond with their students, their patients and their colleagues, and how difficult this was for them; and their perceptions of frequent failures and few successes.

Both in my own institution and in national faculty gatherings, I listened to innumerable stories of how disheartened medical faculty felt. When we asked faculty to write about what kind of person they wanted to be, tremendous idealism and altruism poured out. They described dealing daily with human suffering and wanting to care for patients who needed trusted counsel and empathetic responses to their feelings of powerlessness in the face of illness, and how they struggled to do this within the constraints of a medical system that is often run like a corporate slash-and-burn enterprise, with little time or conscious attention paid to the human needs of those who work in it. The intense interest that I developed in these problems provided the impetus for the research this book describes. I was intrigued by how administrative power was wielded in medical schools and teaching hospitals and by how damaging their culture can sometimes be to the mission of nurturing young, idealistic students and healing the ill with compassion and efficiency.

I wanted my research—both in methods and outcomes—to be congruent with what I sought to have happen in medical education. I wanted our work to dignify the personal and human experience of faculty in medical schools. I hoped that the research would contribute to a transformative movement in academic medicine—fostering a culture of belonging, authenticity, humanism, and vibrancy in learning.

In 2003 I submitted a research proposal with this focus to the Women's

Studies Research Center (WSRC) at Brandeis University and joined that large and amazingly diverse group as a Resident Scholar. Immediately, I was struck by the contrast in the culture at the WSRC as compared to my earlier experiences. During the first weeks, it suddenly came to me that I had never heard the words "feminism" or "feminist" used in a medical school, or in other medical meetings—these taboo words would have been considered provocative or even unsafe in those environments. As I learned more about feminist thinking, I realized that much of the innovation and programming I had implemented over the years was intuitively aligned with feminist principles. Before, I had always felt like an outsider even when quite successful and in positions of some authority, but here I fit right in. I felt so much happier and less stressed than I had in some medical schools. In this congenial, supportive, and stimulating setting, I embarked on my research, and as it progressed, I realized that many medical school leaders would be extremely interested, surprised, and to some degree dismayed by what I was finding out.

The Research Studies

In my first study, focused on the effects of administrative power on women and men in academic medicine, I interviewed a national sample of twenty-two medical faculty, over half of whom were women, and more than a third of whom were women in leadership positions. They were drawn from many different specialties or disciplines and included six basic scientists. They occupied various positions: four were department chairs, one a division chief, and six held deanships. The second interview study was part of a larger action research project, the National Initiative on Gender, Culture and Leadership in Medicine (C - Change) (http://cchange .brandeis.edu). In this project we used a rigorously constructed sample of ninety-six women and men faculty from five U.S. medical schools. These schools had bravely agreed to collaborate to address the stunning lack of women and underrepresented minority faculty in senior or leadership positions in academic medicine. Schools were selected to provide balance in geographic distribution and to be representative of different organizational characteristics of medical schools (public vs. private ownership, NIH research–intensive vs. community-primary care focus). The C - Change project was generously funded for four years by the Josiah Macy, Jr.

Foundation, allowing me to pull together an extraordinary research team of highly accomplished co-investigators.

We selected and interviewed equal numbers of faculty from each of the five schools. Interviewees were categorized by gender, race/ethnicity, department/discipline, and career stage. The four career stages were "early career," those who had been faculty members for two to five years; "plateaued," that is, those who had been faculty members for ten or more years and had not advanced as expected in rank and responsibility; those in leadership roles, such as dean, departmental chair, and center director; and former faculty who had left for a career outside academic medicine. Interviewees were equally divided among the four groups. Participants were research scientists, medical and surgical subspecialists, and generalists. Eighty-three percent held medical degrees (MD or DO), and 17 percent were scientists with a PhD degree. Women composed 55 percent of those interviewed. Seventeen percent were African American/black, and 4 percent were Hispanic or Latino; 20 percent were generalist physicians. Minority faculty, who are present in very small numbers among medical faculty, were overrepresented in the sample, but we sought them out because we wanted to hear their perspectives very clearly.

We conducted one-hour semistructured interviews (15 percent in person, 85 percent by telephone) that were audio-recorded and transcribed verbatim. We asked faculty how they had come to choose a career in medicine, what they had hoped for, and what their values were. We explored when they felt most successful and what barriers they had come up against. We also asked their views on leadership and power and their experience of integrating their work and family lives. The questions were open-ended, nonleading, and unbiased in wording, so the respondent could describe what was personally meaningful and salient.

All the interviewees gave permission for their narratives to be used in research, and in turn we promised to rigorously protect their identities. After repeatedly reading the masked transcripts, the research team identified codes for specific content in the texts (such as "values" and "leadership") and identified themes and patterns in the narratives (such as feelings of being invisible). All the identifying information in the interviews had been masked before we coded the data, and all the names used in the book are completely fictitious.

Although colleagues had questioned whether faculty would be willing to be interviewed, I found from the first round of interviews that when I explained my purpose, not a single person declined. In fact, I was offered more interviews than I could actually manage. Hearing the interviewees' accounts of what was meaningful in their professional lives strengthened my resolve and lifted my spirits. I was continually impressed by the lofty ideals and high standards upheld by these faculty and by their dedication to their work, even when it was overwhelming or extremely stressful. This book distills their stories.

C - Change was not simply a research study but also an action project. It included a Learning Action Network made up of four to six members from each of the collaborating schools, who attended a two-day, in-person gathering held twice a year. At these meetings, people occupying a range of positions within their specific institution, including deans, department chairs, and junior faculty, of different races and genders, learned together and also learned to trust each other in a process that embodied the type of culture change needed in medical schools. The group came together as a community of learners and doers to explore the culture of medical schools, learn from the perspectives of others in the group, and implement practical changes or improvements. The medical school deans and other leaders in this group were more than courageous in volunteering the participation of their faculty and in committing their own time to this priority.

Medical School Structure

There are approximately 119,000 full-time medical faculty (including 34,000 women) in the nation's 131 medical schools. This number has doubled from about 56,000 full-time medical faculty in 1981 as medical schools increased their research activities and expanded their patient care facilities.

For readers who are not familiar with academic medicine, a medical school is an extremely complex organizational culture. It consists of about twenty departments representing different fields of medicine: internal medicine, surgery, psychiatry, family medicine, obstetrics and gynecology, radiology, orthopedics, etc., and the biosciences such as genetics, biochemistry, anatomy, and physiology. The largest and thus most powerful clinical department is usually the department of medicine (that is, internal medicine), comprising many divisions, each representing a sub-specialty: cardiology, gastroenterology, pulmonary medicine, oncology, infectious diseases, and others, each with its own division chief.

Over three-quarters of medical school faculty are trained as physicians. Most (clinical faculty) care for patients and teach medical students and residents (physicians-in-training); some may also have research responsibilities. Twenty-nine percent of faculty are in the so-called basic science departments. These are mostly scientists with PhD degrees, engaged in biomedical research. This group may also do some teaching of medical students, particularly in the first two years of medical school.

Depending on the focus of a department and to some extent that of the medical school, individual faculty spend varying amounts of time doing research. This can be either laboratory research in a basic science department, such as microbiology or genomics, or clinically based research, in which a particular treatment intervention or diagnostic test is assessed for effectiveness in patients. There are also population-based research and health services research, which study risk factors for disease and the delivery of health care, respectively—for example, evaluating the extent to which an intervention is cost effective for a community. A clinical science department faculty member, in addition to seeing patients and teaching and supervising students and physicians-in-training (residents and fellows), often also does research, depending on the emphasis placed on research in that medical school and the type of appointment the faculty member has. Traditionally, teaching and research are required elements of the medical school tenure and promotion process.

The medical school organization is markedly hierarchical. Usually, the most powerful positions are the chairs of the clinical departments because the medical services these departments provide are of paramount importance to the surrounding community, attract strong interest from the local press, and bring in large amounts of money to the institution from billing insurance companies or Medicare/Medicaid. Nonetheless, in the large research universities/medical schools, research scientists are often admired internally more than clinicians, not only because research is considered more intellectually challenging and has the potential of providing revolutionary breakthroughs, but also because the federal government gives the university an additional 50 percent to 70 percent of the grant award for institutional overhead, over and above the salary and other costs granted to the researcher to conduct the research. Departments may compete with each other for institutional money, space, faculty positions, and power, and the protection of these territorial domains sometimes supersedes achieving educational goals—which of course distorts the institution's overall mission.

A Dysfunctional Culture

Our interviewees described a medical school culture that often fails to support the collective ideals and values of the faculty. Faculty were sometimes subject to demands that challenged their ethical and professional standards, and they believed that the organization did not always share their altruistic motives. As a result, they experienced moral distress that not only prevented them from working at their highest potential but in some cases drove them out of their jobs. (Preliminary findings from the C - Change survey indicated that about a quarter of both male and female faculty believed that the culture of their institutions discouraged altruism and that 31 percent of female and 28 percent of male faculty had seriously considered leaving academic medicine in the prior year.)

Interviewees also described a culture with significant problems in how people related to each other. Faculty said they felt dehumanized and unable to trust leaders or colleagues. They felt they did not count as people and that the system encouraged individualistic, competitive behavior rather than collaboration. Dehumanization, dishonesty, and competitiveness led to an erosion of trust in the entire system. It is important to note that in this respect, there was no distinction among different groups; our data analysis showed that these themes were not unique to any gender, career stage, or race and were expressed by faculty in all disciplines. The result is a great waste of tremendous human potential and squandering of public and academic resources.

This lack of healthy human connections in academic medicine leads to an undesirable parallel problem: faculty are likely to treat patients and medical students in the same way they are treated themselves. This has been described as a decline in "humanism" in medicine; its effect is poor communication between doctors and patients, with consequent effects on health care; for example, patients who lack good relationships with their physicians are less likely to adhere to medical advice.

Many of these issues are highlighted in comments by Dr. Francesco, a senior internist who left academic medicine. She pointed out the irony of attempting to train physicians to practice compassionately in an environment that creates barriers to any real interpersonal connection:

> Power in academic medicine mostly comes through money. [For one thing,] the individual at the top has the purse strings. And, somehow, academic medicine has developed this amazing hierarchical structure, which is common to all medical schools. The department chair position has enormous power, which is held tightly for that reason. . . .

> Some divisions report to a department head. The department heads are in some way accountable to the dean, although in many ways the dean is frightened of the department heads because they hold huge amounts of money from their external research funding and clinical productivity. There's a constant balancing and rebalancing of power between the deanship and the department chairs. They are both frightened of each other in some ways. . . . Then in the practice of medicine, you have the attending physician, and the physicians who are less experienced, and then the residents, and then the students.

Dr. Francesco explained that this hierarchical structure was antithetical to the need to create the trust between physician and patient that is required to provide the most effective form of care:

> But [this type of trust and care is] not implicit in the relationship between the deans and the department chairs, or the deans and the faculty. One would hope they have some sense of looking after the faculty, but that's certainly not a widely held concept . . . if the faculty do their work well and work hard, they can stay. But it's not really a culture of "How can we nourish the faculty?" "How can we look after these people?" It's different from what you hold for a patient.

Women's Views as Outsiders

Little has been written about values, power, and relationships within medical schools. There is a modest literature about medical school faculty per se, but women's experience in particular has largely been left out of the conversation. This book presents their perspective, which is in many respects that of an outsider. Underrepresented minority and generalist faculty, who are also sometimes marginalized in medical schools, expressed similar views.

In our interviews, male faculty made the same comments about feeling isolated and lacking connections with their colleagues as did women and underrepresented minorities. They also gave similar descriptions of what inspired them and gave meaning to their work, and their expressions of altruism were as strong as those of women. Although men and women often respond similarly, men still manage to command higher salaries, receive more grants, gain power and status, and get promoted. Women do not. This indicates that although men may indeed dislike the culture of academic medicine, they more readily achieve and are less alienated within the current system. Men do not share the same outsider status as women and do not feel marginalized in the same way women do. What is more, as marginalized outsiders, women do not bear the responsibility for having created such a dysfunctional system. This makes it easier for them—even those who do become leaders—to critique the system as clear-eyed observers and to examine their experiences and come up with practical solutions for the issues that plague the system as a whole. As we will see, some have already succeeded in converting the stigma of outsiderness into positive change. Thus, I use the experiences of women as a gathering of data points and needs assessment that can help drive organizational culture change.

For in fact, we can fully utilize and benefit from the potential contributions of a wide range of people—men, women, and minority groups—only by changing the current distorted medical school culture. This book suggests that women (and minority groups) demand the opportunity to implement their own vision of leadership, using their own, different skills that have the potential to improve medical school culture. In addition to making sure that more diverse voices and perspectives are represented in leadership, we must create a more inclusive, transparent, less hierarchical organization. I believe that this is the most efficient way to address all the problems this book describes. My belief and hope are that understanding the experiences of the women whose voices appear here will enable us to improve the medical system for everyone.

REFERENCES

Pololi LH. Standardized patients: as we evaluate, so shall we reap. Lancet. 1995; 345:966–8.

Pololi L. Career development for medical school faculty: a nine-step planning strategy. Br Med J Careers. 2006;38–9.

Pololi L, Clay M, Lipkin M, Hewson M, Kaplan C, Frankel R. Implementing an academic faculty development course about teaching, modeled on educational theory. Med Teacher. 2001a;23:276–83.

Pololi, LH, Coletta EM, Kern DG, Kiessling LS, Davis S, Entin EJ, Garber C, Opal S, Rakowski W. Developing a competency-based preventive medicine curriculum for medical schools. Am J Prev Med. 1994;10(4):240–4.

Pololi L, Dennis K, Mitchell JA. A needs assessment of medical school faculty: Caring for the caretakers. J Contin Educ Health Prof. 2003;23:21–9.

Pololi L, Frankel RM. Small group teaching emphasizing reflection can positively influence medical students' values. Acad Med. 2001;76:1172–3.

Pololi L, Frankel R. Humanizing medical education through faculty development: linking self awareness with teaching skills. Med Educ. 2005;39:154–62.

Pololi L, Frankel RM, Clay M, Jobe AC. One year's experience with a program to facilitate personal and professional development in medical students using reflection groups. Educ Health. 2001b;14:36–9.

Pololi L, Harris D, Clay M, Jobe A, Hallock J. Institutionalized faculty development program. Acad Med. 1998a;73:9.

Pololi L, Knight S. Mentoring of faculty in academic medicine: a new paradigm? J Gen Intern Med. 2005;20:866–70.

Pololi L, Knight S, Dunn K. Facilitating scholarly writing in academic medicine: lessons learned from a collaborative peer mentoring program. J Gen Intern Med. 2004;19:64–8.

Pololi L, Knight S, Frankel R. Helping medical school faculty realize their dreams: an innovative collaborative mentoring program. Acad Med. 2002;77:377–84.

Pololi L, Lannin D, Mathews H, Mitchell J, Swanson M, Swanson F. The need for culturally based breast cancer education for African American women living in rural North Carolina. Med Encounter. 2000;15:10–11.

Pololi LH, Potter S. Behavioral change in preventive medicine: an efficacy assessment of a physician education module. J Gen Intern Med. 1996;11:545–7.

Pololi LH, Potter S, Garber CE. A competency-based preventive medicine teaching module for medical students. Teach Learn Med. 1998b;10:109–15.

Pololi L, Price J. Validation and use of an instrument to measure the learning environment as perceived by medical students. Teach Learn Med. 2000; 1:201–7.

Putsch RW, Pololi L. Distributive justice in American health care: Institutions, power, and the care of patients. Am J Managed Care. 2004;10:SP45–53.

chapter 2

Women and Medicine: History and Myths

> While the needs and interests of women physicians are inseparable from those of men, they are by no means identical; we earnestly hope and believe that in all questions of family life, with moral and social problems, they will raise the tone, widen the perception and alter the attitude of the profession in general, so as to make it respond more perfectly to the needs of society, and exert a high power for good in all directions. If this be realized, it will be seen that the work of women is absolutely essential and of ever increasing importance and the outlook for this in every respect most helpful.
> —William H. Welch, *Women's Medical Journal*, October 1913

In the eighteenth century, building on the advances in the medical sciences in Europe, American physicians established medical schools and started to organize medicine as a profession. Women, who for centuries had occupied traditional roles as folk medicine healers and midwives, also gradually turned their attention to becoming physicians, and as medical education became more accessible to them, they sought it with increasing frequency. Today, women make up half of all medical students in the United States. A review of the history of women in medicine will help us understand better women's choice of the profession today.

History of Women in Medicine

Over 150 years ago, Elizabeth Blackwell, the first female physician to graduate from a U.S. school (in 1847 from Geneva Medical College in New York), criticized the impersonal nature of medical science in the development of medical careers. To her, and to other early proponents of training women as physicians, medicine seemed a natural choice for educated women, given their family roles of nurturing and caring. Blackwell also argued that having women physicians would address female patients' embarrassment over disclosing symptoms to male physicians. She and similar pioneers believed that women could humanize society and the practice of medicine, promote preventive medicine, and raise the moral tone of the profession. These same values—the importance of caring and the notion that women must be brought in to improve the health care system—are powerfully echoed in our own interviews.

In 1880, there were about 2,000 female physicians in the United States, and in 1900 about 7,000. In 1920, 5 percent of U.S. physicians were women; in 1960, 6.8 percent (out of a total of 229,590); and in 1980, about 11.6 percent (out of nearly half a million). Though women currently make up 25 percent of the 750,000 physicians in the country and about a third of the 119,000 medical faculty in U.S. medical schools, they had to wage a long struggle to become respected as physicians.

Entry into the Profession

American medical schools resisted admitting women on various grounds: women should be in domestic roles; their intellect was inferior; menstruation was debilitating and prevented them from functioning; they had a tendency to hysteria; and so forth. Nonetheless, by the 1880s, six women's medical colleges were in existence. The Boston Female Medical School was founded in 1847, and in 1850 forty women enrolled in the newly opened Women's Medical College of Pennsylvania. The others were the New England Female Medical College, 1856, which later merged with Boston University; Woman's Medical College of the New York Infirmary, 1868; Woman's Medical College of Chicago, 1870; and Woman's Medical College of Baltimore, 1882. In addition, a few male medical schools had accepted women students in response to various forms of pressure. For example, in the late 1880s, four Quaker women—Carey Thomas, Mary Elizabeth Garrett, Mary Gwinn, and Elizabeth King—offered to complete the endowment that Johns Hopkins University needed to survive on condition that women be admitted into the new medical school on the same terms as men. Canada accepted its first women medical students in the 1880s. By the turn of the twentieth century, a number of American universities were accepting women into their medical schools, although the American Medical Association did not open its membership to women until 1915. During those early years in the profession, most women physicians treated mainly children and women.

By 1910 women were nearly 6 percent of medical students, but this figure subsequently shrank because after World War I and the Depression, support waned for women entering the medical profession. Most institutions accepted women based on unwritten quotas, with a temporary increase during the Second World War coinciding with the male military draft. Women did not recapture 6 percent of medical school places until 1950; most medical schools had only two or three women in each entering class. Harvard, to take one example, admitted a maximum of 6 percent women until the mid-1970s.

The women's movement of the 1960s and 1970s encouraged more women to apply to medical schools; in 1969, they were 9 percent of applicants. In 1972, Title IX of the Higher Education Act outlawed discrimination against women with respect to admission, policies, and salaries in any institution receiving federal support; by 1974, women were 20 percent of medical school applicants. During the 1970s, medical schools enlarged their student bodies, and graduates increased from 8,974 in 1970 to 15,632 in 1980. The schools were very successful in removing gender bias from their admissions committees and welcoming women. During the 1980s, the number of male applicants declined, and there were too few to fill the freshman class. Because women applicants met the admissions criteria, by admitting them, the schools could maintain their standards. These changes contributed to the number of women medical students jumping from 10 percent in 1972 to 29 percent in 1980, 39 percent in 1990, and 46 percent in 2000. Since 2002, men and women have applied in equal numbers, and 49 percent of women and 51 percent of men have been accepted; many female students are academically superior to their male counterparts. Since 2004, 16,000 medical students have graduated each year, half of them women, carrying average debts of $150,000.

After graduating from medical school, a new physician chooses a particular field of medicine and applies to a residency program for training in that field. There is an uneven distribution of women trainees across various specialties. In 2007, 37 percent of internal medicine residents; 24 percent of internal medicine subspecialty fellows (such as cardiology, endocrinology, infectious diseases); and 20 percent of surgery residents were female. Among other residency programs, women comprised 60 percent in pediatrics, 46 percent in psychiatry, 62 percent in obstetrics and gynecology, 45 percent in family medicine, and only 7 percent in orthopedic surgery. It is not clear why, but women apparently find certain specialties more appealing, and these choices correlate with the distribution of women medical school faculty members among medical specialties, as described below.

The Struggle for Acceptance

From 1880 to 1930, women physicians played an important role in the nation's liberal reform movements, paying particular attention (as they still do) to the needs of women and children. They found little support for their presence or tolerance of their differences. In 1975, Dr. Mary Howell, a pediatrician and the first female associate dean at Harvard Medical School, restated a belief expressed by nineteenth-century women physicians: that founding a woman's health school informed by "collaborative sharing of effort and responsibility, nurturance, care giving and personal service to others" was necessary to counter the massive resistance of the medical profession to "the beliefs and values held by women for women." She felt strongly that traditional medicine continued to glorify "science and technology to the detriment of face-to-face care giving" (Howell 1975). During her own interview for admission to the University of Minnesota Medical School, the admission officer had told Howell that it would be a waste of taxpayers' money to admit her since she would only get married and drop out of the profession.

In fact, the writings of many nineteenth- and twentieth-century women physicians still sound relevant and modern in their recognition of bias against women. In 1882 Dr. Mary Putnam Jacobi (Jacobi 1882) wrote:

> In this effort, the most serious obstacles to be encountered are not always the most real ones. . . . I ask not, "Is she capable but, is this fearfully capable person nice?" Will she upset our ideal of womanhood and maidenhood, and the social relations of the sexes? Can a woman physician be lovable; can she marry; can she have children; will she take care of them? If she cannot, what is she?

Jacobi founded the Association for the Advancement of Medical Education for Women. She strongly contested the commonly held assumption that women physicians could not function professionally for a week out of each month due to menstruation (in 1875, Harvard University had organized an essay contest on the subject "Do women require mental and bodily rest during menstruation?"). The notion that women were not "hormonally suited to have highly responsible positions" actually persisted into the 1970s (Levin, 1980).

The assertion that medicine is a profession especially suited to women because it alleviates suffering continued through the twentieth century. When women first entered the profession, a widely held concept was that "every woman is born a doctor. Men have to study to become one," as Dr. Ella Flagg Young put it. Subsequently, there were some strong proponents of allowing women into the profession, including Dr. John Bowers of the Josiah Macy, Jr. Foundation (Bowers 1966), who wrote:

> In the recruiting of talent for medicine the feminine half of American brainpower is being ignored. It is quite possible that the need for more physicians can only be met if a larger number of women are attracted to medicine as a career. Beyond the quantitative problem is the fact that women enter fields of medicine such as pediatrics and child and adolescent psychiatry that are in urgent need of physicians. The medical schools and the teaching hospitals should face up to the question. Should there be a higher percentage of women entering medicine? And, if the answer is "yes," as I suggest it should be, these institutions must take positive steps to attract larger numbers of women and make it possible for them to complete the training, including the internship and residency.

In her outstanding book *Sympathy and Science* (Morantz-Sanchez 1985), the historian Regina Morantz-Sanchez notes:

> Early women physicians, like other social feminists, were instinctive critics of the dehumanization inherent in industrialization. They feared the tendency of the capitalist order to turn people into commodities, even as they hailed the positive role of individualism in bringing about female emancipation. Though they misunderstood the place of class and misperceived the roots of economic exploitation, from their vantage point as women

they quickly comprehended that the rationalization of human knowledge could be carried too far. They brought to medicine a critique of the growing primacy of cure over care, and though their values were ultimately lost or swallowed up in the triumph of twentieth-century medical professionalism, this perception, however vague and confused in its articulation, formed the basis of their criticism of the profession to which they so fervently wished to belong. In the present decade, some feminist scholars are again boldly challenging the ideological assumptions of the professional elite by suggesting that male and female values differ and that the professional world would benefit from an infusion of female concerns.

As later chapters will explain, we found in our interviews indications of the differing values Morantz-Sanchez refers to, suggesting that women can still bring valuable new perspectives to medicine and health care.

However, in contrast to those early women medical pioneers, women physicians were mostly silent in the women's movement that began in the 1970s. They usually conformed to the prevailing mores of the profession without taking on decision-making roles or authority within the male-dominated system. Nonphysician scholars like Morantz-Sanchez described what they saw as the pressures for women physicians to be shaped by the prevailing culture of medicine. They pointed to a shortage of empathy and a responsiveness to the dominant achievement standards, rather than an attempt to change these expectations and incorporate more humanistic qualities. As described in Chapter 6, women medical faculty still recognize these problems today, and they still often keep their opinions to themselves; instead of attempting to change the system as a whole, they create microenvironments, such as small working groups, where they can find sympathetic collaborators and some relief from what they see as, at times, a dehumanizing culture of academic medicine.

Where Women Stand in Academic Medicine Today

Women now have equal access to medical school education and have graduated in sufficient numbers to be well represented in senior faculty and leadership positions in the nation's academic medical centers. Yet, despite the large cohort of well-trained potential female leaders, women have not advanced to positions of authority as expected. In fact, the situation has hardly changed since the mid-1980s. Even in 1980, 30 percent of medical students were women; if they had moved normally through the system, many would be leaders now. Instead, the vast majority of full professors are still men: the average medical school has 188 male (21 percent) and only 35 female (4 percent) full professors; only 17 percent of all full professors are women. Women rarely sit in decision-making positions in medical schools, teaching hospitals, research institutes, or professional organizations. Only 8 percent of clinical department chairs and 13 percent of basic science department chairs are women. This means only one or two in each school; sixteen medical schools have never had a female department chair. There are only eight women deans among the 131 U.S. medical schools. All these figures reveal that when medical students look for role models of success, they rarely see authority figures demonstrating the possibility of high achievement by women. The Association of American Medical Colleges maintains both an extensive database and website that document demographic trends in U.S. medical school faculty and students (aamc.org).

Women faculty also tend to congregate in certain fields. In Internal Medicine and its subspecialties they are 30 percent; in Pediatrics, 45 percent; in Obstetrics and Gynecology, 45 percent; in Surgery, 14 percent; and in Orthopedic Surgery, 12 percent. In Internal Medicine, only 14 percent of full professors are women, even though 30 percent of all faculty in these departments are women. In Pediatrics, 24 percent of full professors are women, in Obstetrics/Gynecology, 18 percent; and in Surgery, only 7 percent.

It is also interesting to examine the unequal distribution of high-ranking women among academic medicine departments. In the clinical science departments (for example, Internal Medicine, Surgery, and Pediatrics), only 10 percent of women faculty become full professors, compared with 28 percent of male faculty (AAMC 2008). These figures have remained largely unchanged for over twenty years. In basic science departments (e.g., Physiology, Molecular Biology, Anatomy), the numbers are somewhat better; 24 percent of women scientists become full professors, compared to 42 percent of men).

These differences are surprising. Why should women fare better in basic science departments than in clinical departments? One might expect women to excel in clinical care because of their empathy, nurturing, and self-organizational and multitasking skills. It is not clear why so few women achieve leadership positions in clinical departments, but one possible explanation may lie in the fact that clinical faculty have opportunities to acquire great power. These departments bring in more income, partly from research grants but mostly from treating patients and billing insurance companies for costly procedures and encounters. Another source of power is that outstanding clinicians are lionized in the lay press more often than basic scientists. Our interviews suggest that women are not fully part of the culture in clinical departments, meaning that they lack the personal and professional connections that help people move into leadership and acquire power. A third factor may be that these departments are run more hierarchically than science departments, and—if the distaste expressed by our interviewees for the arbitrary exercise of power is any indication—women seem not to thrive in such environments. In any case, this unexpected distinction suggests that the reasons for women's failure to rise to positions of authority can be discovered not by examining specific characteristics of women, but by looking at the culture of academic medical centers.

Why Women Have Not Advanced: Four Myths

Four reasons are commonly proposed to explain why so few women become leaders in medical school faculty: they are distracted by the need to care for their children, which impacts their professional performance; they leave the faculty early in their careers, so they do not remain in the system long enough to be promoted; they simply have no ambition to be leaders; and they need to develop certain skills to make them equivalent to men. However, examination of the facts reveals these notions to be myths.

Children as a Distraction

The standard explanation for women's failure to be promoted to high positions is that their children prevent them from focusing on their careers. One suggested solution, therefore, is to provide child care. But this explanation is not satisfactory. Although having children makes it more difficult for women to juggle family and career, this is only one of the factors at play; nor does it explain the fact that women beyond the child-care years and those who do not have children do not become leaders either.

Despite preconceptions among both the general public and many scholars, women physicians are slightly more likely to marry than women in general (U.S. Census 2000). Since the 1980s, the marriage rates of women physicians have been slightly lower than those of male physicians, but significantly higher than for women in teaching and law. Most women physicians are in dual-career families (and in 1980, half were married to physicians). Women physicians are less likely than other women to divorce, and they have children at rates comparable to the rest of the U.S. population. Other studies showed that single women and married women scientists without children did not publish more than women scientists with children, and that the academic rank achieved by women physicians did not correlate with the number of children they had (Graves 1985; Cole 1987). These data contradict the assumption, in reports and opinion pieces attempting to address the issue of leadership, that for women in medicine, work and family roles conflict more than in other professions.

One study of women physicians who graduated from Yale University School of Medicine between 1922 and 1998 found that 61 percent were married or partnered, 30 percent had never married, and 10 percent were divorced. Forty-nine percent had children, 11 percent had no children and were not planning to, and 40 percent did not yet have children but intended to. Forty-two percent of the women with children had them during medical training, and 58 percent had them after starting practice (Potee et al. 1999). A 1997 AAMC study showed that women were more likely to have their first child during or before residency training than later in their careers (AAMC 1997).

Studies comparing women to men who entered medical school at the same time show large differences in advancement. For example, one study that surveyed a national cohort of medical school faculty members found that after an average of eleven years in a faculty position, 23 percent of men but only 5 percent of women achieved full professorship, even when taking into account hours worked, specialty or productivity differences such as grants, and numbers of publications. The researchers found no significant difference in numbers of children among female and male faculty at advanced ranks (Tesch et al. 1995; Tesch and Nattinger 1997).

Devotion to children is quite evident in our interviews, but women readily go on to speak of their need for a rich professional life; their connection to their children does not decrease their dedication to and excitement about their careers. Dr. Door, who practiced medicine and did research, summed up her dedication to her work and her family, feeling that she managed both quite well.

> Dr. Door: I like to be doing a lot of things at once, so sometimes I would be covering the floor, I would [also] see patients down in the clinic because they want to see me, and sometimes I would cover one of my colleagues for the clinic. You would be doing a million things at once—you're doing okay. Not to forget that I have three kids of my own and I'm married. I just feel like, oh my God, you're managing it all, you're making a good life for your children, you're taking care of your patients and you're getting great cases, and you're learning. That's what I would say when I feel at the top of my game. . . . I always say my greatest work is my children, and the regrets I have are not being there for everything. Because I'm taking care of a lot of other people's children. It's a juggle, and my children have had to learn over time that Mommy has to go to work, but what I try to do when I come home is really spend that quality time and plan to do things with them when I do have the time off. My husband and I have worked out a situation—we're basically a team. If I'm here doing this, someone has to be home, if we're not going to hire somebody, to make sure the kids get to point A, B, C for their activities. It's a juggling game of managing with your partner and communicating who is going to do what task and give your kids quality care when you're there.
>
> I honestly feel, even though I haven't been there all the time, I've still watched them grow under my eyes. I feel like I'm an example for them—three kids, and I have all girls—that you can achieve what you want to do, you just set your heart there and that the things that might give you bumps along the road do not have to interfere with your goals. Your career is to be strong, not dependent on a man. I feel like I'm that example for them. I feel really good about that. Furthermore, if I was at home, 24/7 with my kids, I would just be nutty. I'm a better person coming into the situation after I've been away than if I'm there all day long.

The research literature agrees that medical women find their multiple roles extremely rewarding, experiencing work and family as mutually enriching and beneficial (Shrier et al. 1993; Shrier 2003; Barnett 1998; Barnett and Rivers 1998). All this evidence suggests strongly that women do not fail to advance because of having to choose between child-rearing and medicine.

Attrition

A 2007 analysis by the Association of American Medical Colleges (Alexander and Lang 2008) shows that women medical school faculty do have a slightly higher attrition rate compared with men. Looking at cohorts of faculty over a ten-year period, we see 43 percent of women faculty, as opposed to 37 percent of their male counterparts, leave academic medicine. At the first-time assistant professor level, these figures are 45 percent and 43 percent respectively—which means that most attrition of men and women occurs early in their careers.

In any case, since overall, only slightly more women than men leave academic medicine, the claim that they are not in leadership positions because they do not remain on the faculty long enough has no substance. The proportions of men and women who remain on the faculty are actually very close. Yet the women advance much more slowly—or not at all.

No Ambition for Leadership

There is a widespread notion that women faculty do not aspire to leadership. Women are said to have more limited aspirations and to lack ambition. For example, Anna Fels, a psychiatrist and faculty member at Cornell, maintains that women and men have different attitudes toward ambition: women too often "seek to deflect attention from themselves," often shunning credit and shifting it elsewhere. They also change their behaviors by becoming more demure when competing directly with men (Fels 2004). Neither of these actions is surprising, given that research on women leaders has shown that women are less liked when they behave like male leaders and are penalized for assertiveness.

Even people who have studied why women do not advance in medicine will say that women faculty do not seek leadership positions. But this assertion is quite contrary to my own experience, as well as to the results of our interviews, as Chapter 7 will show. I suspect that these people are mistaking women's modesty for lack of ambition. Their mistake may be compounded by the fact that women dislike the egotism, self-aggrandizement, and sometimes manipulative behaviors they observe in many current leaders in academic medicine and make efforts not to behave this way.

Rosabeth Moss Kanter, a distinguished expert on management, showed clearly in her book *Men and Women of the Corporation* that women's roles in organizations and their lack of presence in leadership positions are linked to the organizational culture and the lack of opportunities it offers them. Women adapt their aspirations for leadership to what they perceive is available, Moss Kanter says; there is no gender difference in aspirations (Kanter 1993). Our medical faculty survey results similarly show no statistical difference in the proportions of women and men who would like to be in leadership positions.

Lack of Necessary Skills

Another common approach in the attempt to address the lack of women in leadership is a "skills deficit" model, based on the assumption that women lack the skills necessary for success. The idea is to train women in the same skills that men use to succeed, such as assertiveness, negotiation, and leadership strategies. Once their failings are "fixed" by equipping them similarly to men, women will become "successful." Embedded in this concept is the notion that these skills, which men already have, are the ones needed to produce "success." It is also frequently said that one reason women lack needed skills is that they do not receive adequate mentoring.

Although women would certainly benefit from developing their skills in many areas, so would men. And although it is true that women lack mentoring, that too applies to men; research shows that only a small proportion of faculty overall receive effective mentoring. Preliminary results in our survey show that 37 percent of women and 43 percent of men are satisfied with the mentoring they receive. (Prior national studies have shown that about a third of medical faculty report being mentored in some form.) In our survey, about half of male and female faculty agreed that they "get the help I need with how to advance in my career." More fundamentally, this approach ignores the possibility that different forms of leadership such as those that women might introduce could instead be an improvement. After all, both medical education and health care in general are systems with massive problems that can use fresh ideas and new perspectives.

Our own examination of women's reasons for becoming physicians and scientists, and of what they find most inspiring and rewarding in their work (described in the following chapter), demonstrates that these myths are just that and have no basis in these professional women's actual lives. There is, in fact, nothing wrong with the women. Instead of repeatedly bringing up their supposed deficits, we should turn our attention to changing an imperfect and outdated system so that it can benefit from the very real skills that women possess in abundance.

Why Women Choose Medical School

What do women seek when they choose a career in medicine? This is an important question, since half of new physicians are women, and as more women become leaders, their aspirations will help to determine the development of education, research, and clinical care in the nation's medical schools—and thereby the course of health care.

When we asked women faculty why they chose medicine, the main themes that emerged were that they had loved science in high school and college and wanted to use it to help people.

> Dr. Silverman: Choosing medicine was not really a surprise. I don't come from a family of physicians, but it's something I always gravitated to . . . I love the sciences and it seemed to just follow. But during college I weighed whether I should do something more like marine biology or environmental biology, and I realized I loved being with people. The animals weren't going to do it for me. And after that there was never a doubt in my mind, to go into medicine.

> Dr. Grant: Before I went to medical school, I was going to get a PhD in biochemistry. But I felt that medicine was a place where you would help people, whereas science was meeting your own need for the excitement of discovery. And yet medicine was fantastically interesting, because you learned about the biology of disease. So my interest in biology as well as my altruistic leanings were met by going to medical school.

Dr. Harwood: At one point as an undergraduate, I faced a fork in the road: Did I want to pursue zoology, wildlife biology, that side of things, or did I want more of a biomedical focus? And I settled on the biomedical focus because it seemed more helpful. It would just make a bigger difference.

This combination of intellectual curiosity and altruism, developed early in their lives, persists throughout the careers of such women, motivating and sustaining women faculty through what are, as we will see, some problematic aspects of medical school culture.

REFERENCES

Alexander H, Lang J. The long-term retention and attrition of US medical school faculty. Analysis in Brief, 8(4), Washington, DC: AAMC; 2008.

Association of American Medical Colleges. Medical school admissions requirements 1997–98. Washington, DC: AAMC; 1997.

Association of American Medical Colleges. Faculty Roster 2008. Available at: http://www.aamc.org/data/facultyroster/.

Barnett RC. Toward a review and reconceptualization of the work/family literature. Gen Psychol Monogr. 1998;124(2):125–82.

Barnett RC, Rivers C. She works/he works: how two-income families are happy, healthy and thriving. Cambridge, MA: Harvard University Press; 1998.

Bowers JZ. Women in medicine: an international study. N Engl J Med. 1966;1: 362.

Cole JR, Zuckerman H. Marriage, motherhood and research performance in science. Sci Am Med. 1987:256;119–25.

Fels A. Do women lack ambition? Harvard Bus Rev. 2004;82(4):50–60.

Graves PI, Thomas CB. Correlates of midlife career achievements among women physicians. JAMA. 1985;254;781–2.

Jacobi MP. Shall women practice medicine? North Am Rev. 1882;134(302):52–76.

Levin B. Women and medicine. Metuchen, NJ: Scarecrow Press; 1980.

Howell M. 1975. A woman's health school? Social Policy. 1975;6(Sept/Oct):50–3.

Kanter RM. Men and Women of the Corporation. 2nd ed. New York: Basic Books; 1993.

Morantz-Sanchez R. Sympathy and science: women physicians in American medicine. New York: Oxford University Press; 1985.

Potee RA, Gerber AJ, Ickovics JR. Medicine and motherhood: shifting trends among female physicians from 1922 to 1999. Acad Med. 1999;74:911–9.

Shrier DK. Psychosocial aspects of women's lives: work, family and life cycle issues. Psychiatr Clin North Am. 2003;26(3):741–57.

Shrier DK, Brodkin AM, Sondheimer A. Parenting and professionalism: competing and enriching commitments. J Am Med Womens Assoc. 1993;48(4):122–4.

Tesch BJ, Nattinger AB. Career advancement and gender in academic medicine. J Irish Coll Physicians Surg. 1997;26:172–6.

Tesch BJ, Wood HM, Helwig AL, Nattinger AN. Promotion of women physicians in academic medicine. JAMA. 1995;273(13):1022–5.

U.S. Census 2000: United States Profile. US Census Bureau web site. Available at: http://www.census.gov/prod/2002pubs/c2kprof00-us.pdf.

chapter 3   What Inspires and Motivates
             Women Medical Faculty?

> I consider myself to be among the fortunate of the earth. I cannot imagine a life
> that could have brought me more satisfaction. Doctoring yields enormous per-
> sonal gratification precisely because what I do benefits others.
> —Carola Eisenberg, MD, former Dean of Student Affairs
> at Harvard Medical School

As women's careers developed and they began to recognize their professional opportunities, their motivations remained remarkably similar to
those that had led them to go to medical school—and that motivated the
pioneer women physicians 150 years ago. Our interviewees' early, sim-
pler, and more general aspirations became more specific as they matured
and discovered how their ambitions could be deepened, focused, and fulfilled through real-world practice. In response to our queries, women
described in strikingly passionate and idealistic terms what in their work
inspired and energized them.

Variety and Complexity

One dominant theme was that, as Dr. Door stated in Chapter 2, women
loved the variety and complexity of academic medicine. They *wanted*
diverse, complicated, and changing responsibilities. Many spoke of the
richness of being able to see patients as well as to teach and/or do research. Dr. Conrad, an internist, said:

> It's the investigation, thinking about how things work, trying to figure out
> the parts that you don't understand or don't know. That's in research

and it's also in patient care. You are trying to put yourself in this person's head and body and figure out what's going on, and I don't make that much distinction. I guess that's an MD approach to research. So I'm thinking the same things when I'm out taking care of a patient as I am when I'm in the lab.

Dr. Flower, a primary care physician, explained that her responsibilities for patient care and biomedical research complemented each other in a particularly fulfilling way.

Dr. Flower: With my grant and on my project, I travel usually at least one day a week around the state. I have clinics. I have hospital inpatient duties. I do some work with the med school in terms of teaching. I did some work out in the community. I just love the variety of what I do!

Dr. Rigoni, another internist who in addition to patient care conducted laboratory research, described how these different responsibilities complemented each other.

I guess there are different high points depending on what's going well and what's not going well. In research, the more academic part of my job (I do basic science research in a lab most of the time), when you have a hypothesis about how a certain compound or experiment is going to work and you do the experiment and you get an expected result, or even when you get an unexpected result, it tells you something about biology, you can see how it could be applied to patients and treatment. . . . You think you're a very small piece of the puzzle; you can see where this could fit into a bigger picture of how diseases work and how people could be better treated. It's very exciting and stimulating, and it pushes you toward saying, "I should keep moving forward with this train of thought or this kind of investigation."

And then, conversely, there are days or weeks when experiments aren't going well. But there may be times in the clinic when somebody says, "I really appreciate what you did for me" or "I'm feeling better because of that medication you recommended." And that energizes you when the research isn't going so well, and you think, "I just have to keep plugging along and sooner or later, that part of things will pick up again."

Professor Booker, a nationally prominent basic scientist at a prestigious university, became quite animated as she explained her perspective on the intensity of the scientific process and how she enjoyed integrating research with training students. She described the complexity of what she was trying to accomplish and how she achieved her scientific advances through interacting with her students. The combination of the science and the intellectual pursuit, together with nurturing trainees, were what made her work so exciting.

> Dr. Booker: So when a project is going well and it's hard and there's some breakthrough, it's a combination of you and the people you work with—in my case they're post-docs or graduate students, and a few undergraduates—it's very stimulating, because you're learning new things but also you're learning with other people. Training them. You can see them coming along. You are turning them into scientists; that's the process. And it happens at a different pace for everybody. But for every student you are successful with, it becomes exciting at some point. And it's not only the process of educating, it's that I'm deeply interested in the projects. But whether they work or not depends on the interaction between me and the students. I don't do experiments myself, so if I can't somehow get them excited, it doesn't work.

Caring for Patients

Many physician faculty found clinical care deeply satisfying and considered themselves fortunate to enjoy the profound rewards of helping a patient. Dr. Kern, an internist, said:

> Probably the most satisfying thing in my work is when I get some positive feedback that I've helped someone deal with a serious illness or helped them recover or they express thanks for help I've offered them.

Women spoke of the deep satisfaction of knowing a person and being trusted—being in an almost sacred space with the inner and outer world of another human, a living, feeling, acting person. They described "seeing and feeling into the problems" in a patient's life and said how meaningful it was to "make a difference" in people's lives, to "participate in patients' lives in a significant way." This sense of reward extended beyond curing disease and treating medical problems to "caring for people" and "helping them die." For example, a specialist in geriatrics said:

> Dr. Cole: I take care of the frail elders. That really energizes me in a way that I can't explain. I love these people. I love my nursing home residents. Even after I leave [the teaching hospital] at the end of the day I can go to the nursing home even though I'm tired, and it will re-energize me. . . . You are more often than not looking at caring over curing, because these people are at a point where you are not going to cure anybody, but you can provide them and their families with a lot of care.

Faculty felt a deep involvement with and respect for their patients.

> Dr. Peterson: There is a lot of personal satisfaction and fulfillment in helping parents with their children. And then if their children are sick, in helping the children themselves get better. That's a bit of a charge for me.

> Dr. Cole: I wake up in the morning and I say, geez I have the best job in the world because I take care of patients that I care about, that I find interesting and find the work intellectually stimulating.

> Dr. Schmidt: Recently I had a family experience with severe illness and death, and being on the other side of it, seeing what a poor job [the physicians] did, and how the subtlest things a physician did were of incredible comfort to the family, it really made me look at my own practice differently. Now, amazingly, I was able to find solace in my practice during this time period, and actually looked forward to being with patients. Even when my mind was somewhere else, or I was worried with this particular situation, I found that one way I could deal with the impact was sitting one-on-one and continuing to see patients and trying to be just a little bit better than I had been before.

> Dr. Francesco: Over my career, I've been very moved by the enormous trust that a patient can place in a physician and the privilege the physician has of holding that trust. It's like a sacred space. It is a place for trust. I believe that students and physicians need to understand that this

is their privilege, and how unusual that is, and what an enormous responsibility that is. And also, how rewarding it is as a physician to be able to enter into that relationship, that intimacy with someone that would generally take many years to develop—if you ever developed it—with a friend, or even a partner or family member. It is comparable to family.

Exhilaration of Scientific Inquiry

As suggested by the many women who saw scientific discovery as integral or complementary to their roles as caring physicians, women faculty enjoyed research immensely.

> Dr. Rose, a senior pathologist: Originally, I didn't seem to know what I wanted. As I got deeper into research, I found it exciting and energizing, and I think that's clearly why I stuck with it.

> Dr. Victor, a basic scientist working in a clinical department: Initially I went to graduate school—I wanted to study public health. I could have worked in the pharmaceutical industry. I tried. I went to a company and worked there for a while and realized it's too focused on profit, and I was more interested in studying what really lit my fire, rather than what lit profits. I couldn't think of a job where I could do that other than academic medicine.

These women found intense intellectual stimulation and excitement in constructing research questions and doing scientific work that revealed new insights into our understanding of life and disease. Seeing their own discoveries translated into clinical applications gave them great satisfaction. Along with this came the thrill of having their ideas and new knowledge receive external recognition and accolades upon publication in scientific journals. They saw this as a legacy of their hard work, intellect, and contribution to the biomedical sciences.

Women relished the complexity of being in a continuous learning process, where they were continually building on their own knowledge and skills, while integrating new information. Intellectual freedom and autonomy were particularly important to them; indeed they reveled in the expectation that they could do anything they liked, expressing deep appreciation for this great good fortune.

Dr. Rose: The things I liked about it: the intellectual rigor of it appealed to me, the freedom appealed to me. . . . You can think about a complicated problem, in this case, a medical problem, and try to find a solution, and as long as you can convince somebody else that you're finding a solution to an important problem in a useful way, you can really do whatever you want. It gives you tremendous intellectual independence. I can sit down and think about how a particular disease works, and think about experiments I might do that might contribute to solving that problem. As long as I can convince other people that those ideas are good, I can probably get money to actually see if my ideas are correct.

Dr. Victor: I enjoyed the science and I enjoyed trying to understand the biology of disease and how it worked in populations. And I probably could have been practicing someplace else but I like the research aspect, and in academic medicine you can do research on the topic of your choice.

Generally, these women thrived on the constant intellectual challenge and rigorous standards of research and learning. The complexity of disease, managing patients, and evidence-based research requires continuous questioning of science and one's own thinking—especially in a competitive research environment where getting funding requires intellectual rigor and persistent hard work.

Dr. Anthony: I get to choose the questions I want to work on—and I hope they're good questions and I get funded—and then I just love the other people. It's very stimulating to be surrounded by lots of interesting, smart people who are all working on the same goal. So, again, it's the variety and the intellectual stimulation.

Dr. Harwood: The few moments when I realized that I was figuring something out that people hadn't figured out before, that I was seeing data no one had ever seen before because my experiments had generated it, and I was going to get to interpret it, and it was mine! [laugh]—that was pretty exciting.

Dr. Victor: I think it's developing the [research] hypothesis, reading around the science and trying to understand the biology and marry that with observations. The fun part is when I'm observing a phenomenon, for example, esophageal adenocarcinoma, that seems to be increasing so rapidly and affecting white people—and white men. Then trying to think, what is it about them that is different? Just thinking through the hypothesis, what they could be exposed to—that none of us are—and coming up with a question that I then write a grant about; that is what really excites me!

In addition to publishing their research, faculty also described their relief and excitement at receiving funding for it, particularly from the National Institutes of Health (NIH). NIH funding is the main and most coveted source of support for research in academic medical centers. NIH (and other federal) grants provide the most generous funding for overhead costs, most of which goes to the university, which reciprocates by giving more recognition to the researcher. Such funding is increasingly difficult to get, since more and more researchers are seeking it at the same time that NIH budgets are diminishing. It is also gratifying to receive funding because writing proposals is not only arduous and time intensive, but largely unfunded work.

Making a Difference

Beyond the sheer thrill and anticipation of discovery, women said they valued research for its potential to help people, emphasizing its applications to illness or social issues. They enthusiastically articulated a desire to combine the altruism of medicine and the excitement of research. Dr. Rouge, a PhD working in a clinical department, and Dr. McGuire, an anesthesiologist early in her career, both commented on the rewards they felt from applying science and discoveries made through research to patient care. Dr. Rouge focused on the care of patients during rehabilitation and Dr. McGuire on patients (or "cases," doctor-speak for "patients") during surgery.

> Dr. Rouge: My initial aspirations involved two parts, teaching and clinical work. I discovered in my masters level clinical work that an awful lot was not known about how people recovered. I was working with neurology patients, and I found that people were recovering, but not necessarily in proportion to what we understood as the organic damage. I would

ask my supervisors and the neurologist, "What's going on here . . . why are some of these people doing so well and others not?" and they would say, "Well these are the mysteries of the recovery process." And I felt, as a scientist, that this was not a good enough answer, that we ought to be able to figure out what was going on . . . and offer that to the patients who were not doing well, and hopefully encourage their recovery. That's part of what started me on the way to my doctoral work—recognizing how little was known about something I thought was so important.

Dr. McGuire: I have felt really energized when I have had a challenging case: when you really have to understand a lot of basic science and your intervention [discovered through research] can actually make a difference in the outcome. And to have it go well, especially when you're doing that with a research fellow; you have an opportunity to teach while you're doing it. I find that to be very gratifying.

Dr. Rossi, a basic scientist, also found the translation of her field of science to clinical settings very motivating.

I find it really fascinating that what I do might have some sort of translation to the clinic. I was never very much excited about basic science in the sense of studying *Drosophila* or *C. elegans* or yeast because it was very hard for me to get my mind around why this was interesting and what kind of applications it could have. I love and am fascinated by what I do because of its application.

Faculty often alluded to the mission of higher truth that can be pursued in academia in contrast to the profit motive or expedience that they believed was often the main motivator in industry.

Dr. Marissa: Intellectual independence, I love the science. I'm curious, I want to find answers to biological questions that we have here. I'm excited by this . . . versus industry.

Improving the System of Medical Care

Faculty also talked about wanting to "make a difference" in a broader way.

Dr. Ireland, a senior physician: For me, being at a place like this aligns totally with what I thought I would be doing with my life, which is trying to make the world better through health care.

Women felt that the variety of roles offered by academic medicine represented a unique opportunity to combine different interests, all related to improving the practice of medicine as a whole. They eloquently described wanting to become leaders in order to advance biomedical research and improve the way medical schools operate, including their schools' approaches to clinical care and training. Dr. Sanders, a senior internist, and Dr. Goldsmith, a senior surgeon, both described this clearly.

Dr. Sanders: I think it's the ability to really make a difference and make a change, and you can do that in a number of different ways. You can do it in a basic research lab or you can do it running a clinical lab, making sure that diagnostic tests are accurate and bringing in new technology. You can do it running a division with the same sort of basic goals: How do I make this a good division? What can be transformed, what will be the outcomes, or what are the desired outcomes? How do I get there? I really enjoy that kind of thinking.

Dr. Goldsmith: Being able to change the culture of how we take care of patients, the whole paradigm of involving the patient and the care team work [referring to "patient-centered" care, which includes patients' perspective and opinion in decision making]: those things are exciting. Making medicine even better than it has been in the past is probably the most exciting thing now that I'm an administrator more than a surgeon, even though I still operate and see patients.

Advancing the Health of Vulnerable and Underserved Populations and Women

Whereas many interviewees identified "helping people" as a motivation to enter the medical profession, later in their careers some focused more specifically on advancing the health of the underserved and of women. Before entering the profession, they were not familiar with the concept of people being medically underserved and did not realize that there was unequal access and provision of care for some groups of people – often defined by race or low income. Once they encountered this reality, their generalized altruism shifted to a more sophisticated view of academic medicine as providing the opportunity to address these problems. This opportunity was often the reason they chose to stay in academia.

> Dr. Sanders: My commitment is to advance the health of both women and individuals of color.

> Dr. Geordino: I didn't have aspirations for a career in medicine to begin with, but putting a first husband through graduate school, I saw the readily available health care for the folks in that community that we didn't have in [our own region]. That was my "Aha" moment. I wanted to do something to improve the access and the quality of health care here. Only later did the concept of actually going to medical school come up, when the medical school was developed here. From that time I was just kind of seeking ways to do that.

> Dr. Cooper: I really hoped to make a difference in terms of changing the way women with ovarian cancer were treated, of improving survival and quality of life for them as they underwent treatment. I was very interested in women's health.

> Dr. Schmidt: Stemming from my years at medical school and a lot of volunteer work I did, I think my heart really was in helping underserved populations.

These comments reflect the fact that the medical work of many women has highlighted previously unaddressed issues. Studies show that female physicians are much more likely than men to focus educational or research efforts on women's health issues. Before 1985, medical textbooks relied almost exclusively on male physiology and men's biological reaction to diseases, even though women's physiology and response to disease and treatment are different. Women were often not included in clinical research studies, so it was simply assumed that the results applied to women also. It was female physician scientists who fought for inclusion of women patients in research studies and led the field in women's health studies. As female scientists began studying illness in women, previously poorly understood gender differences, such as in heart disease, were better elucidated, and different symptom patterns were recognized in women, resulting in earlier diagnosis. Female physicians are also more likely to integrate into their practice preventive medicine and health promotion, a field of medicine that has been neglected for years (Beaudoin et al. 2001).

It was as a result of the efforts of women physicians such as those quoted here that the government authorized public funding directed at women's health. The Office on Women's Health (OWH) was established in 1991 to improve the health of American women by advancing and coordinating a comprehensive women's health agenda throughout the U.S. Department of Health and Human Services, focusing especially on the millions of underserved women in America.* The National Institutes of Health founded an Office on Research on Women's Health in 1990 to serve as the focal point for women's health research at NIH and to ensure that women's health research is part of the scientific framework of NIH and throughout the scientific community. This Office also ensures that women are appropriately represented in biomedical and biobehavioral research studies supported by NIH.

Teaching and Nurturing Juniors

Another major theme among interviewees was a deep love of and passionate commitment to teaching medical students and residents. As part of the faculty development programs for medical faculty I created in North Carolina, one of whose goals was enhancing teaching skills (see chapter 1), we asked faculty to write an answer to the question: "How would you like to define yourself as a teacher?" The responses we received were quite moving (Pololi et al. 2001; Pololi and Frankel 2005). The quotes below illustrate the meaningfulness our faculty derived from their professional activities and their enduring aspirations. The faculty writers were anonymous.

---

*The National Centers of Excellence in Women's Health, funded through the OWH, were instrumental in promoting research and implementation of programs addressing women's health care in the United States. The Office on Women's Health also established four National Centers of Leadership in Academic Medicine with the goals of mentoring medical faculty for career advancement. I was the founding director of one of these.

I entered this profession to try to minister to others through the blending of caring and science. I am at a point of transition in that I feel humbly comfortable that I am able to help others provide for their health needs; however, I feel a tug to pass on to those coming behind me those values, attitudes, and content to charge them to care for the sick. In other words, to the sick I feel a sense of duty to transmit the tools of caring and science to the next generation of these clinicians who are privileged to care for them.

I would like to become someone who facilitates learning and growth in others. I would want to create learning environments where we all, learner and teacher/facilitator, feel supported and respected. Within that environment I would like to meet learners at their learning edge, help them define what they want to learn and help them through that process of learning. I wish to be open to learning from my learners and to their perspective. There will be no place for shame or humiliation in the learning environments I create, and learners will grow to take responsibility for their own learning. I will be operating within a community of learners where the admission of lack of knowledge is welcome and seen as an opportunity, and where good intent is assumed in all. Care will be taken of the emotional, physical and personal, as well as the intellectual, needs of the learner in my learning community.

In much the same way, teaching was a driving motivation for our interviewees as well. They positively reveled in the relationship of teacher and learner, sinking deep into the mystery of helping another person move from feeling ignorant to feeling competent and excited by learning. Faculty loved seeing this excitement in their clinical students and research trainees and felt deep satisfaction when these students succeeded—as though the students' success shone a light on themselves as teachers and mentors. Thank-yous from students had lasting impact.

Medical training takes the form of apprenticeship, which means that almost all medical faculty have trainees assigned to their clinical service. Women who taught in conjunction with other roles, especially clinical care, considered the educational part of their work especially meaningful and important.

Dr. Barkman: . . . another reward is when someone like myself, who is, I would say, not a dedicated teacher—I'm not here strictly to teach medical students—when a student says, "this is really very exciting, I was never able to put this together before." That is very rewarding.

Dr. Schmidt: I have felt most successful when I see or talk to a resident who is just so excited about some program we were able to get them into, and see the wheels beginning to turn about how they might actually use this in their future—they are going to be a cardiologist or a primary care physician—when I see them get excited about something we were able to bring to them that they didn't have three or four years ago.

Dr. Westenfelder: From the age of nine I had decided that I wanted to be a physician, I don't know why. . . . I'm the first one in my family to even go to college, with no one else in health care. And from the very beginning before I even knew what academic medicine was, I knew I wanted to teach medicine because probably as much as I am a physician, I am a teacher at heart. So, when I went to medical school, I never considered private practice, it was with the intention that I would stay in academic medicine. Probably the reasons were a love of teaching but also wanting to be where I thought I would have the greatest intellectual stimulation.

Dr. Peterson, a pediatrician, described education as part of the intellectual stimulation of her work:

Having an opportunity to continue to learn things. To explore new information, new strategies, like getting into education. I get a charge working with the younger doctors who are just learning about the world of medicine and are in an accelerated growth phase. Watching them change—three years isn't a long time, but they change so dramatically from when they walk into the hospital as interns to when they leave, because they have to go out into the world to actually be doctors. The same with the medical students. We see them in the third year and some of them come back to us a year later and they're almost like different people. That's a bit of a charge for me too—having the opportunity to facilitate people's personal development in this field.

Basic science faculty also derived profound gratification from teaching.

Dr. Rossi: When I was a post doc, what I found successful was experiment work when I'd uncovered a very exciting finding. Now what I find successful is when my students, my post docs, can get their experiments to work and they find something interesting and novel. I really look more toward the people in my lab being able to succeed, rather than myself.

Dr. Risen: I have a research lab and I'm responsible for PhD students. It's being part psychologist and part babysitter. I try to carefully recruit students—I don't always look for hotshot students, I try to look for students that have something in them that needs developing. I think that's what turns me on.

Many women focused on innovation in medical education. They talked of their excitement at achieving through education the larger goal of influencing health care:

Dr. Venetia: [The reason] it was so enjoyable and meaningful was that I felt I was having a positive impact on larger, larger issues, larger world. I could influence how and what medical students learn, [and that] would have an impact on how they practice. So by extension I could have an impact on people's health and well-being. It sounds kind of grandiose, but having that connection to a larger issue is really important to me. When I was thinking about ways to incorporate attention to relationships in health care, I felt that area can have a major impact on the culture of medical education.

Dr. Schmidt: I love the teaching. We work very closely with agencies that provide careers for homeless in the city. I've been volunteering with them for years, and now I am getting my residents out there. To see the residents get excited about something that I'm excited about, and that's good for the community and for people who really don't have access to care, that's what really gets me. But it's not didactic or typical ward-attending kind of teaching; it's broader teaching about the world of medicine in the community.

Dr. Tonder: What I loved was creating curricula, thinking about how to do things better and differently for students in ways that would promote more effective learning environments and a curriculum that more accurately reflected the skills they needed as clinicians, both for physician assistants and docs, and that was really challenging.

Interdisciplinary Collaboration

Collaborating with a group of colleagues in different disciplines or a variety of backgrounds, with the shared purpose of improving research or clinical outcomes, was another extremely motivating experience. Women loved the opportunity that collaboration afforded to move outside their own discipline.

> Dr. Venetia: That work gave me an opportunity to meet and work with a whole host of people across a variety of institutions who were all working on a common project and shared some common concerns, and that was a wonderful thing. I worked very closely with faculty across a number of departments in the medical school and also a bit across disciplines with nursing and pharmacy faculty. That was very energizing.

Dr. Jones, a medical subspecialist, collaborated in writing a research grant proposal with colleagues from different departments. She explained that this was very helpful in addressing the challenges of grant writing.

> What I liked was working with people from different backgrounds, coming together to work on a common problem. The other people made me think of things in a way I hadn't before. And they were people I was able to hand pick . . . for being very thoughtful people. . . . That project involved a lot of intellectual energy, had an outcome, a grant—a product that was really a challenge to produce.

Several common themes run through the quotes presented here: women faculty derive meaning and fulfillment from a variety of interests and activities; they seek to have a broad, significant impact, whether in medical education and training, the application of research, or healing patients; and an important value that permeates all these different areas of their work is the ability to create a heartfelt connection to patients, colleagues, and students.

Given the tremendous satisfactions described by these women faculty, it is hardly surprising that the vast majority persist in their careers and do not leave the profession. For the most part they lead rich professional lives in medical schools, and the system provides sufficient personal reward for them to remain. Yet our interviews also made it clear that there are many serious problems in the academic medical environment that have driven some to leave and prevented those who remain from achieving their full potential and making the greatest contribution they are capable of. The following chapters will explore these issues and investigate the untapped abilities and perspectives that women can bring to bear to improve the health care system as a whole.

REFERENCES

Beaudoin C, Lussier MT, Gagnon RJ, Brouillet MI, Lalange R. Discussion of life-style related issues in family practice during visits with general medical examination as the main reason for encounter: an exploratory study of content and determinants. Patient Educ Couns. 2001;45:275–84.

Pololi L, Clay M, Lipkin M, Hewson M, Kaplan C, Frankel R. Implementing an academic faculty development course about teaching, modeled on educational theory. Med Teacher. 2001;23:276–83.

Pololi L, Frankel R. Humanizing medical education through faculty development: linking self-awareness with teaching skills. Med Educ. 2005;39:154–62.

chapter 4

Relationships and the Human Condition

> { ... the salvation of this human world lies nowhere else than in the human heart, in the human power to reflect, in human modesty and in human responsibility.
> —Václav Havel, Speech to the U.S. Congress, 1990 }

We need physicians who are compassionate as well as competent. Both scientific knowledge and also the ability to create personal relationships are central to providing effective health care (Suchman et al. 1998). A growing body of evidence suggests that self-aware physicians are more effective, satisfied, and efficient in providing care, and that caring, empathic physicians have patients who are more satisfied and more likely to follow medical advice (Novack et al. 1997). Thus, the basic tasks of medical schools are to nurture trainees' self-awareness and emotional development and to help students, faculty, and medical practitioners learn how to form caring, healing relationships with patients and their families, with their communities, and with each other (Tresolini 1994).

Extensive research has found that medical students become less altruistic and empathic during medical school; however, little research has explored academic medical culture's effect on medical faculty, who should be the models of caring and compassion for their students. In our interviews, most women and men reported a lack of connection to their colleagues and even said they were treated at times quite shabbily by some of them. They described feelings of dehumanization, erosion of trust, and a sense of being invisible and isolated within an environment where competitive individualism was rewarded and collaboration undervalued. A lack of truly collegial relationships, and especially the absence of trust, creates significant barriers to professionalism and productivity.

This chapter describes how this sometimes "toxic" culture creates barriers to good relationships, as viewed through the experiences of the women we interviewed. Our data show that the way medical schools are structured and the norms of behavior among faculty can create huge barriers to effective relationship formation. The interviews often depict a medical school environment that could at times negatively impact patients and our system of health care as a whole.

Failures in Personal Relationships

Problems with personal interactions in the academic medical culture emerged as a central theme in our interviews. Although we did hear very positive comments about teaching, about relationships with patients, and in some cases about supportive, collaborative relationships with close colleagues, the majority of interviewees described negative perceptions of personal interactions. This was true even though we asked open-ended questions, for the most part sought accounts of positive experiences, and did not request accounts of problems with personal interactions. Comments about relationships tended to arise spontaneously rather than be elicited by the interviewer. Although this book is focused on the experiences of women, in fact, both women and men spoke similarly about relationships in the interviews.

Disconnection

Two fundamental worrisome experiences in academic medical culture were a sense of disconnection and having few trusting relationships with colleagues and supervisors. Many faculty members, at all career stages, described feeling isolated and lacking nurturing relationships. They felt that the norms of their environment and the way it was structured did not value or support relationships. A number of faculty commented that decision makers felt distant from them, whereas those in positions of power also said they felt disconnected from the faculty generally.

> Dr. Tonder, senior faculty: I realized that I valued relationships and interpersonal behavior that the institution did not. . . . So a lot of what women do to make a culture more nurturing—help people grow as

human beings, become, in my judgment, better clinicians—is not something the institution values. They can do it if they want, they get all kinds of laudatory praise, but they do it on their own time.

Dr. Tonder felt that often when faculty and trainees came together (whether in administrative settings, clinical settings, or teaching), there was no time devoted to nurturing people as individuals rather than just dealing with the task at hand. Her comment implies some hypocrisy, since the institution (for example, in the person of a department chair) might say that it wants to nurture people but in fact did not place sufficient value on this goal to devote funded time to it. From the institution's point of view, a faculty member who spent less salaried time nurturing relationships could be bringing in additional income by seeing more patients or writing more grant proposals.

This failure to foster work relationships contributed to the sense of chronic disconnection pervasive in the interviews. Linda Hartling, a scholar at the Stone Center at Wellesley College, describes environments that "discourage or suppress the conditions that facilitate the development of growth-fostering relationships; that impede mutual empathy, mutual empowerment, movement toward mutuality and authenticity" as cultures of disconnection that diminish people's energy for their work and make them feel disempowered and confused (Hartling and Sparks 2002). Indeed a number of women faculty expressed a sense of confusion regarding this culture, even though they were very capable and highly motivated. As Dr. Venetia put it, "It's a very difficult system to negotiate because things are not as they seem."

Competitive Individualism

Interviewees described an intensely individualistic, competitive environment where rewards usually went to individual accomplishments. Respondents perceived that individuals and institutions tended to function on behalf of their own self-interests, making decisions and choices that benefited themselves rather than contributing to the common good—and sometimes came at the expense of the common good. As one interviewee put it, "the system is set up to perpetuate itself." It was accepted that a stressful and competitive environment was necessary to promote scientific progress and achievement. That is, the system is designed to create barriers at all levels to collaboration and collegiality. For example, credit and promotion result from being first author on research papers, not from being part of a group responsible for a collective achievement. An interviewee commented on the effects of such a system:

> Dr. Reed: The first question out of people's mouth is "Well, what is this going to do for me?" "What paper do I get out of it; where will my name come in the list of authors?" "Who's looking out for me" and all that stuff. And it's just like there should be enough to go around.

Respondents often linked the competitiveness of climbing the academic ladder to the development of aggressive, self-seeking, and uncollegial behavior on the part of faculty who previously had not acted in this way. Dr. Tonder, noted:

> There were colleagues of mine to whom power meant a great deal, and I watched them become people I didn't like as they dealt with this hostility and grabbed for the power. They achieved a great deal, and I don't take it away from them, but in the course of it, they lost their humanity. They became people I could no longer respect. They became dishonest and manipulative, and I just wasn't willing to go there. . . . I just wasn't going to go to one more meeting and sit there and feel abused.

A number of faculty suggested that coping in the medical school environment brought about this change not only in colleagues but also in themselves. A senior subspecialist, Dr. Ireland, described the "toxic" environment of the division meetings of her department. Such a meeting might discuss administrative issues or interesting clinical cases.

> The environment was quite toxic in an interpersonal way. It was actually quite threatening to my emotional survival. I never felt safe in that group. . . . I felt very little support from almost everybody. They were so mean. Language-wise, I could just never keep up with them, but I did learn. You learn to become extremely aggressive and obnoxious. I found over time that it hurt my soul to be that mean. I tried to detach from

being like that, but the environment was like that. It wasn't just compromising my values, I would have to swallow so much unmitigated grief.

If you exposed a little bit of yourself, showing some vulnerability, it was played upon on some level. And the last year or so that I was in the group, I almost never talked when I was in the division meetings because I was so worried about having someone twist my words around. I realized that in that environment I had become a person that I didn't really want to be. I really needed to find some way to detach from that.

The truth was, if you weren't willing to act as if you were superior to everyone else in the organization and to treat people like crap, being really mean on ward rounds to residents and medical students—if you weren't willing to make them feel badly, and if you acted like doing that wasn't OK—then you were attacked verbally, you were undermined. They tried to undermine my ability to get my work done. If you were to talk to the unbelievable number of faculty who have left that division over the past fifteen years, not a single one of them would tell you they felt safe there.

Dr. Ireland, adapted, but at a cost: "My assumption would be that a lot of their behavior was from a place of insecurity in which they learned some really powerfully negative pushback behavior that I learned too"— for example, attacking others to shield their own sense of vulnerability.

Dr. Skinner, another woman in a leadership position, explained that she was not naturally sufficiently "cutthroat" to function well in such an environment. To describe what she meant, she used the image of a rating system from 1 to 9:

One is the kind who will shoot his mother for something and 9 is the kind who can't kill a fly. I get 9's and I've been told, "You've got to be more toward a 5." But you know, I like me as a 9. It makes me a very good friend, but it is not great for academic medicine. For academic medicine, [you need to be] somewhere between a 2 and a 6—on the cutthroat side—because don't let anybody fool you: everybody is cutthroat in this business, only the currency is different, and women don't do well in that setting only because we have no training in that. We have no exposure. I have sons, but if I had a daughter I'd make her do some kind of team sport. Not because of teamsmanship, but because they've got to learn, people will do dirty, creepy things to you and the playing field will be totally uneven and you still have to get out there and do it. . . . It always shocks me how people double-cross each other. They can be so nice to each other, then at another meeting—that is very hard for me to deal with, but that is academics. You've got to make nice to people you hate. You have to make nice to people who step all over you to get wherever they want, and that's a lesson I don't think I'll ever learn—and that's something that hurts women.

Another possible result of this competitiveness was what interviewees described as a "heroic model" of personal over-extension. Faculty felt it necessary to present themselves, and be observed, as being present and working hard for very long periods of time.

Dr. Jones: They [faculty members] have to prove how busy they are and so they stimulate this cult of busy-ness. If you are looking relaxed or you're caught reading something in your office, you're obviously not busy enough. It's a culture of tornadoes; you have to act like a tornado in order to prove to people that you're really working hard and you're so busy you can't possibly do one more thing. This is all you hear about . . . how busy people are.

Dr. Harwood: One of the things I didn't like was this whole culture that my friends and I used to joke about, that we called "macho science." It was all the braggadocio about how many hours you spent in the lab last week, and when was the last time you saw your wife and all of that stuff. It was not about productivity, it was about how much time your face was at the bench or at your desk.

Dr. Jones: The supermom phenomenon, the cult of busy-ness, I think that drives wedges between people too. You always have to appear busy. What room does that leave to say, "I went and saw the gardens today, they're gorgeous."

A number of faculty found the self-promotion required by competitive-ness and the heroic model distasteful. One woman noted, "She [her supervisor] said, 'You have to brag, you really do.' And that's very difficult for many people because it's not the nature of some of our cultures, experience, and maybe just family culture, too." Dr. Sanders, a senior woman, summarized the environment as a "marketplace":

> You have to position yourself so that you are part of the decision making. You can't expect and wait to be the beneficiary of benevolence . . . the recipient, and so I guess that's been my guiding principle; this is a marketplace environment. Even though we like to think we live the life of the mind, in fact it's a marketplace and you have to have something to bring to the table that gives you equality.

Undervaluing People's Humanity

Numerous faculty complained of not being recognized as a person beyond their professional role. No attention was paid to what people were feeling, and there was no invitation or expectation that they express their emotions or talk about important personal issues related either to work or their personal life. Faculty said this refusal to engage them as individuals had a depersonalizing effect. The culture seemed to ignore the qualities that made them able to address human needs and show compassion and sensitivity to others. Dr. Jones, a midcareer subspecialist said:

> Nobody cares what makes me tick here. I'm completely invisible—as a human, as a person. A nonprofessional person. It just seems like I go through most of my day with nobody recognizing who I think I am. Or acknowledges me in any complex sense . . . or me as a unique individual. I just appear to be what I represent.

Dr. Harwood commented: "Check your humanity at the door, that was how it felt. Any sign of—this is gonna sound harsh, but—any tendency toward kindness was viewed as weakness."

Being unable to bring one's authentic feelings into the workplace has a dehumanizing effect. Thus, several interviewees asserted that being ignored as individuals prevented them from being fully present in their work life, since they brought only selected aspects of themselves and their thinking to their professional lives. Some faculty feared being penalized for discussing problems at home and said that it felt risky to talk about personal or family problems at work. Dr. Barkman, an early career basic scientist, said:

> Our son came home and announced his girlfriend was going to have a baby. You know, those are life events that come with the territory, and they are big things that you need to share with your colleagues at work. But there's always a concern that it's going to be used against you because they're going to realize that you are distracted or not functioning as you do normally. There are a few people you can let your guard down to, but it's a risk.

Another faculty member described what happened to a colleague:

> Dr. Plant: It was tough, I happen to know that he had a very ill child. And I've always thought that somehow that would increase your capacity for empathy, but it doesn't necessarily. In his case, as far as I could tell, the effect of it—not necessarily his intention, but the effect—was to close him off rather than open him up. So he wasn't able to bring the piece of him suffering because of his sick child to his work.

Disparagement and Disrespect

We found little indication that medical schools cultivated appreciation of people's efforts. Rather, the focus was on finding fault. Researchers, educators, and clinicians spoke of feeling disrespected or of not being valued as faculty who had contributed to the medical school's successes. Dr. Jones commented:

> People tend to defend their territory, defend and assume that you're attacking them. The assumption is that people are trying to think ill of you. Or are trying to find the moment where you slip up. Who wants to work in that kind of environment?

Another dimension of disrespect was the perception that the organization was not loyal to the faculty. Dr. Risen, a senior basic scientist, commented:

I think what they've done recently, not to me as much, but to faculty who have always had grants and who are now having trouble getting them. . . . If people can't get grants, they're making them feel bad, making them feel worthless. I think that's not nice. And instead of saying, "Good job, you've done a good job. You've gotten grants for 20 years and you've been a good teacher. . . . Now [they say instead] you don't have a grant, now you're worthless."

Numerous faculty members noted that their contributions were not recognized by the medical school. For example, Dr. Schmidt remarked: "We're not rewarded by the medical school at all. A few people each year might be recognized, but for the ongoing day-to-day grind, we're not recognized by the medical school for our efforts." Many others said that education was not considered important; one remarked on the obvious "devaluing of education. That's what I'm all about, and that's clearly not what the medical school is about."

Erosion of Trust and Truthfulness

Two social theorists, Seligman and Luhmann, define trust as an individual's belief that he/she can rely on the sincerity, benevolence, and truthfulness of others (Luhmann 1979; Seligman 1997). Fugelli, a Norwegian physician and professor who has written about trust in health care, describes "two types of trust, personal and social trust. Personal trust is the trust that you have in an individual (such as a spouse, friend or colleague). . . . Social trust is trust in societal institutions; for example the government, the military or a health care system" (Fugelli 2001). An essential element of trust is the belief that an individual or an institution will act in your best interest—an important factor in enabling you to feel safe. This basic belief in the institution or in colleagues was rarely expressed in our interviews, although many physicians commented on their own efforts to create this feeling and belief with patients. Because they lacked trust in colleagues or leadership, some faculty said, they were unwilling to express an opinion for fear of retaliation. Dr. Carter, a plateaued faculty member explained:

The hardest thing for me was to be in a department where you couldn't express [your opinion] without feeling that you were jeopardizing your career. The hardest thing was that I wasn't honest to myself sometimes, because I was afraid earlier on that I would lose my job—I would get kicked out of the department. I don't know if that would have happened, but it did happen to other people. There were people in our department who lost their jobs over their being expressive. Their lives were made absolutely miserable.

Dr. Cole, a midcareer faculty member, explained that she overextended herself out of fear that if she was not seen to be working so hard, she might lose her job. She expressed no trust in her supervisors, no sense that they might help her rather than find fault with her.

> Early on, when I was doing purely clinical, I was bringing in more money than anyone in my division, partly because I would be working until ten o'clock at night and just thinking, "These people may fire me. I've got to do all this work. You know, I can't ever refuse anything." So I was really, really, really killing myself, and of course, getting older and feeling more and more tired.

Another very significant problem that may be partly related to the erosion of trust in the culture of medical schools is the high levels of ethical misconduct reported among federally funded faculty researchers. Martinson, in a landmark 2005 research report published in *Nature*, surveyed over 3,000 early and midcareer scientists who were funded by NIH and asked them to report on their own ethical behaviors in research (Martinson 2005). Overall, 33 percent of respondents said that in the previous three years they had engaged in at least one of 10 unethical behaviors such as questionable relationships with students or research subjects, using others' ideas without permission or credit, not properly disclosing involvement in companies whose products were based on their research, changing the design, methods or results of a study in response to pressure from a funding source, falsifying or "cooking" research data, inappropriately assigning authorship credit, and inadequate record keeping. The authors comment, "little attention has been paid to the role of the broader research environment in compromising scientific integrity . . . certain features of the working environment of science may have unexpected and potentially detrimental effects on the ethical dimensions of scientists' work." Recently, government agencies and professional organizations such as the National Academy of Science have focused on responsible conduct in research, but in this quest they have not looked at how the culture of the biomedical sciences might affect scientific integrity.

Data from our interviews illustrated similar problems. Respondents described breaches of academic integrity that seemed to be tolerated by their administrations.

> Dr. Schmidt: I work on projects, where if I present any kind of tantalizing evidence someone down the hall will go and do those experiments and scoop you and essentially take all your ideas and just run with it, because they're bigger and they're faster. It's also stealing of ideas. You know, you send a grant to have a colleague look it over and lo and behold your data ends up in their grant.

> Dr. Barkman: What he had a wonderful ability to do is to take all of my hard work and give himself credit for it.

Having good relationships with colleagues and feeling less vulnerable and competitive in terms of resources and stability in the organization may help scientists hold onto their integrity and do work they can be proud of without feeling that they are incurring too much personal risk.

Still another issue of trust involves leadership. Dr. Tonder recalled administrative dishonesty:

> My chairman asked me to take over the new faculty. He would give me things I was supposed to tell them we were going to do for them. I would say to him, "We don't do this for people. How can I tell people this is available when you and I both know we don't follow through on that?" He said, "You have to because that's the only way they'll come here." Well, I don't lie. That's not what I do.

Dr. Geordino, a midlevel administrator, described angrily how, in the past, her own department chair had lied to her in a similar way.

> The lowest point in my academic medical career was when I found that my department chair had lied to me when I came to join the faculty. And that he seemed to feel perfectly OK about doing that.

I know this sounds ridiculously naïve, but he had been my advisor previously and he recruited me. He told me that because in my specialty you
normally don't take patients with you when you go, I wouldn't have to
sign a restrictive covenant. My husband had a job which didn't pay very
well at that time, and we really were strapped for finances. When
he put me on the faculty, we decided to buy a house and try to get into
it before the first of the year to help with income taxes. So I went ahead
and started working, and my chair said not to worry about the restrictive
covenant. He said, "We'll take care of that." I worked for a month and a
half, we bought a house, and then he said, "Oh by the way, you've got to
sign a restrictive covenant." I said, "You told me I wouldn't have to."
"Well . . . too bad." Basically he knew that the practice group wouldn't
allow that. But he had lied to me about it. I said, "What other options do
I have?" "Well," he said, "[you] just don't get paid." I wouldn't have gotten paid for the month and a half to two months of work that I'd already
done. Finding out that he had deliberately put me in an untenable position [was] kind of a low point in my career. Right after the high point!
Which was getting out of residency and feeling so powerful and smart.

The issue of dishonesty emerged in the educational enterprise too. Dr.
Tonder said:

> We would tell students they were going to get excellent teaching, but
> they kept increasing the number of patients that the doctors had to see,
> and I watched the education of the students falling off everyone's radar.
> I said, "We're lying to the people who are doing our evaluations, we're
> putting things on paper that we don't do, and we're not being fair to the
> students." It was like: "We have to make money so the students are
> going to have to suck it up." And what happened was that the people
> who were the best teachers ended up leaving over and over again.

She too eventually left academic medicine for a community practice even
though she had been a highly successful and respected leader in her field.
   Being able to trust one's leaders is key to effective leadership and
thereby to the effective functioning of an organization. For example,
James Macgregor Burns, in his seminal 1978 book *Leadership,* empha-
sized the importance of relationships to what he called "transformational

leadership," which raises both leaders and followers to higher levels of morality, motivation, and performance. Inability to trust one's leader thus can have profound negative consequences for individual faculty and the medical school as an organization.

The following extended interview excerpt is a particularly disturbing description of an extremely untrustworthy culture. Dr. Venetia was a highly successful and well-respected medical faculty member who left academic medicine because of the type of dissatisfaction she describes here. She connected her experiences to the existence of financial difficulties in the medical school—what she called "a resource-restrained environment," something fairly common in academic health centers.

In a resource-restrained environment people are very worried about their own positions in an institution. I think that changes the rules for some folks. They feel that somehow they have to preserve their own position and so feel justified in doing whatever to solidify their position. A culture that allows that sort of thing to happen is a puzzle to me, and I don't have a way of explaining it. I think that is partly what makes being in that kind of culture so very stressful. You have no one to explain people's behavior.

It reminds me, some years ago I worked in a federal prison as an instructor, and walking into that prison was like walking into an alternative reality, into an alternate culture where words meant different things, and behaviors signified different things. In many ways the medical school culture is a lot like that. There are all kinds of strange social structures and interactions. It's hard to figure out your place and your relationships, it's hard to know when you react to something if you're reacting to what someone else really meant or [laugh] if you're reacting to what you think they might mean in any other circumstance. It's a very difficult system to negotiate because things are not as they seem, people are not straightforward.

The similarities are that in both circumstances there are always lots of secrets and a lot of agendas that are not spoken and not made overt. People are always reacting and engaging with one another on a lot of different levels, with different people at different times and in different circumstances not being fully cognizant of the whole story, ever. So you can get yourself into trouble very easily by saying something that sieves into some other scenario that you're not even aware of. That can come back later and be used against you, or misinterpreted. Everyone is interpreting things in light of what they know, which is different from what everybody else knows. It's very, very difficult to negotiate a culture like that, 'cause you just never know where you stand with anybody or how something you say could come back to haunt you in some other circumstance.

For example, in the medical school I had a supervisor I had to report to, discuss things with, be open to about problems that needed solving. Initially I was very open in talking with her, for example, about difficulties with staff members. I would go to her and say, "About this situation with so-and-so, this has happened, and how would you suggest we handle it?" This kind of information was used, unbeknownst to me till much much later, to undermine my entire office and operation. . . . For example, she would report these issues to her supervisor in a way that was not about solving a problem. It was about, "This is a bad situation and we have to get control of it and take authority away from them in all these areas because of these really bad problems." In fact in most cases, the problems were short-lived. Her agenda was to take this information and use it to control rather than to help, and to undermine rather than to help. And I didn't know that. I thought that our relationship was one of support—that she was there to support me. And so I was talking on one particular plane and she was talking on a totally different plane and using it in various other ways.

And similarly in the prison, people would come to you and tell you something or I would tell somebody else something, and they would take that and use it in various, sometimes very nefarious ways [laugh]. I would be totally unaware. You end up feeling so incredibly naïve, but of course why would you ever suspect? It seemed like there was no end to what was possible to suspect. I was continually surprised, in *both* institutional settings, about the extent to which things were not as they seemed, and people were not as they seemed. It's an incredibly stressful way to live. In fact, if I had to say which was more stressful, I would say the medical school, because you know with criminals you expect a certain amount of that pathology [laugh]. You don't expect it when you're dealing with colleagues—and that's the thing, they were not colleagues; they behaved in exactly the opposite way. Just last week a colleague who also left the medical school here told me that it took her about three months after she left to start, as she said, thinking normally again. She likened it to battle fatigue. She said it's almost like posttraumatic stress disorder. That you have to teach yourself to live in a normal world again.

Interviewer: You describe a tremendous betrayal of trust.

You couldn't trust your own colleagues. Certain colleagues, yes—for example, the people in my office. We trusted each other fairly implicitly. We would get burned every once in a while by somebody who turned traitor and ratted on us or whatever, but we tried to maintain it. It was an island of normalcy, where we could be honest with one another and share some values and work straightforwardly on projects and ideas. It was the only thing that kept most of us from going totally bonkers.

Interviewer: You said earlier, when the funding gets tight, somehow that changes the rules. Are you saying that one rule that's changed is about truthfulness and ethical behavior?

Yes, I think that's probably the case. I was a little bit removed from the clinical academic environment, being in medical school administration, but I wonder sometimes if that kind of behavior is considered, in some cases, to be business as usual. In a typically male environment, for example, is there typically this dishonesty, or maybe not just total dishonesty, but withholding of information, and the intrigue that goes on, the competitiveness and so on. Is it always there, just intensified when resources are tight? Maybe when the money is flowing and everybody gets some there is less competition, maybe there's always this underlying culture or way of doing business that just isn't apparent until resources are tight.

Here you have a profession that's supposed to be about caring. It just strikes me as so antithetical to that, it makes me wonder how people who behave in that way can ever deal honestly with their patients. I have in mind a person who is also a big clinical researcher, has a lot of federal grants, heads up a lot of programs. I get the sense that he has that competitive edge all the time, I'm not sure if it's just in times of constrained resources.

I agree with Hartling that negative relations can be barriers to faculty vitality, creativity, and satisfaction. Like Dr. Venetia, many of our faculty described serious trust problems that impacted professionalism and productivity, to the point of sometimes driving them out of academic medicine. Certainly, our interviews demonstrate a mismatch between the prevailing approach in academic medicine and the expectations and aspirations we saw women faculty bring to their work in the previous chapter. At the very least, such problems make medical schools much less supportive and positive workplaces than they could be. Worse, since the existence of the behaviors described by our interviewees is antithetical to fostering superior patient care, biomedical research, and educational excellence, these problems can undermine the fundamental goals of these institutions.

Successful Relationships

Relatively few faculty described good personal relationships with their colleagues. When positive relationships were present, such connections seemed to have important protective or buffering effects against the dysfunction of the culture overall. Dr. Barkman said:

> We have a small group of junior faculty who have been thrown together into each other's laps by all the turmoil, and that has been a wonderful thing because we can say, "Oh my gosh, this project or line of thinking isn't working out. There's basically something wrong there and I can't figure out what it is." If I were to say that to a senior colleague, I would put at risk their evaluation of me because I had made such a grave mistake, so identifying those colleagues can help you sort out the problems you have at work.

Research shows that physicians remember for decades mistakes they have made, feeling guilty and humiliated and isolated in their shame. Only by creating transparency, so they can discuss mistakes openly, can these destructive feelings be relieved. Equally important, open discussion enables the physician and others to learn from these mistakes and prevent them from recurring. These findings are reflected in another comment by Dr. Barkman. When asked how her aspirations in medicine were being fulfilled, she replied:

> I guess with establishing relationships in the workplace of trust, relationships in which I can howl my failures without fear of retribution in some way, so that part is terrific. To work in an environment doing something that you like to do and having colleagues around you who are for the

most part supportive or a number of them, that's very rewarding. I still don't know if I'm going to succeed . . . so that's a scary or uncomfortable position.

Respondents valued particularly their research collaborators. Dr. Stevens, a senior scientist who had left academic medicine said, "I felt very little sense of belonging except to my own research group, which felt like a team with a wonderful mix of people."

Positive Relationships with Students and Patients

Numerous faculty spoke of rewarding, valued relationships with medical students, residents, and patients. Particularly gratifying were interactions with physicians-in-training:

> Dr. Grant: The sense of belonging I had was at its highest when I was with learners. I never felt a particular kinship to other faculty as faculty. I think it was pretty much when I was immersed and surrounded by students that I felt like I was a member of the university.

Many faculty spoke of their high regard for patients. Establishing trust in their relationships with patients was very important to them.

> Dr. Francesco: The final outcome is trying to form this trusting relationship between the physician and the patient. So that the physician can be responsive and helpful regarding the patient's suffering. And of course there is a lot of power in that relationship too, the physician has enormous power, and the patient has very little power, and most patients feel that power differential. On the other hand, the primacy of the patient and the whole professional ethic is that the physician will hold in trust the patient's well-being, and never compromise that.

> Dr. Peterson: I like my patients and I like watching them grow and I like watching them work through problems and come out on the other side in a positive light.

> Dr. Cole: One woman, whenever she came in, continued the saga of her 12-year-old granddaughter whose mom got her involved with a 28-year-

old man because her mom was a drug addict. My heart would break for her. And people telling all sorts of stories that were just amazing to me, but this was their life and sometimes, when they came in, that, I think, was what it was for, to have someone to talk to.

Dr. Coleman: I have mostly worked with underserved communities, so these are not academic mentors, but just extraordinary patients that I've met in the workhouse, schools, and homeless shelters who have shaped my view of life, but they have not been faculty.

Relationships with Collaborators

Some respondents described collaborations with a few colleagues that created a very supportive environment for research and education.

Dr. Anderson, a senior internist: I really try to make a collaborative environment where everybody feels that they're part of the decision making and part of effective change . . . it's a much better environment if there's collaboration and support.

Dr. Risen, a senior basic scientist: It's great when it happens, but when it happens, it's because you're sitting with somebody at lunch and talking about your work and you think, "Oh, I work on that. Let's do something together . . . I've gotten a grant by doing that". . . . You go to meetings; you go to each other's seminars. And so several of us collaborate on that, but it's not because anybody told us to. It's because we found each other. Collaboration is the best thing.

Dr. Francesco derived tremendous gratification from creating programs for faculty that facilitated relationship formation, programs her faculty valued greatly. She remarked that it was collaborating and forming relationships with other faculty members that gave her the feeling she belonged in the institution:

I was there for a sufficiently long time, had enough people go through our programs that I think there was some sort of penetrance in the school. I remember, as I was leaving, realizing that I could walk down the very long corridor between my office and the cafeteria, and many of the faculty I met had participated in those groups and would greet me in a warm way. That felt very nice, as it hadn't always been easy to do that work and get it established in the school.

Why Relationships Matter

A considerable body of research explains why a fearful, disconnected culture—such as described by the quotes above—can have widespread negative effects. Quantitative studies by other researchers describe some findings similar to the picture that emerges from our interviews. A 1995 study of U.S. medical faculty showed that they were less satisfied in every aspect of their professional life than those asked similar questions in 1986. A 2006 survey of four U.S. medical schools found elevated rates of depression and job dissatisfaction, especially among younger faculty. In this survey, 20.5 percent of faculty reported symptoms consistent with clinical depression, with women reporting slightly higher levels of anxiety and depression than did men (Schindler et al. 2006).

In the survey of four schools, basic scientists reported small but significantly higher levels of job satisfaction than academic physicians, and in general, being married mitigated some of the negative effects of the academic environment. The majority of respondents indicated that their initial job expectations were not being realized, they were not the contributors they used to be, and that their productivity was decreasing. Significant numbers felt unsupported. Such high levels of physician dissatisfaction are additional evidence pointing to dysfunction in the culture.

A major problem among physicians is burnout (Revans 1996; Spickard et al. 2002). As investigated in rigorous studies by Maslach and Leither, burnout involves a distinct set of psychological attributes: emotional exhaustion, depersonalization, and a decreased sense of accomplishment, which they describe as "an erosion of the soul." The researchers found burnout in this sense to be particularly common among health-care professionals (Maslach 1982). In the 1999 Physician Worklife Study, which surveyed 6,000 physicians, female physicians were 60 percent more likely than male physicians to report signs or symptoms of burnout (McMurray et al. 2000). This research group found that burnout was higher in women physician groups, particularly in academic medicine, where it was linked to lack of control over one's work. A 2003 report by Shanafelt and colleagues found that 37 percent to 47 percent of academic faculty experience burnout (Shanafelt et al. 2003). A recent study in the Mayo Medical School found that of 550 faculty in the department of medicine, 43 percent of women and 31 percent of men met the criteria for burnout (Shanafelt et al. 2009). Burnout is related to less autonomy, more administrative work, less time with patients, less NIH funding, and balancing the demands of patient care, research, administration, education, and family life. In our own survey of faculty in academic medicine, we found that 48 percent of women and 41 percent of men said they felt burnt out. Fifty-four percent of women, and 48 percent of men, had considered leaving their institution in the past year. It is clear then, that something must be done to support both men's and women's emotional well-being.

It must be acknowledged that even though we realize that relationships affect patient outcomes, and we know that there are problems in forming these relationships, we do not know how much of this difficulty results from current fiscal constraints. These factors may be beyond the control of leaders to fix. However, there have been no studies of factors that prevent (or encourage) these relationships from being created. Our study is an attempt to begin doing this.

Positive Relationships and Patient Care

Relationships among people working together are important in all fields, but interpersonal relationships seem particularly relevant in the medical workplace because the primary purpose of academic health centers is to care for patients. Indeed, considerable research shows that connection and communication between physician and patient are important for the patient to develop a therapeutic relationship with the doctor. The literature confirms the importance of trusting relationships between physicians and patients for improving patient care and clinical outcomes.

Medical researchers' use the word "humanism" to mean respecting the patient's viewpoint, attending to his or her psychological well-being, regarding the patient as a unique individual, taking into account the patient's family and social environment, and demonstrating warmth, compassion, and empathy. Hauck showed that patients were more likely to stop smoking if they perceived high levels of humanism in their physicians; they were also more satisfied with their physicians (Hauck et al.

1990). Another body of research indicates that doctors give better care when they are aware of their own feelings and reflective about their responses to patients and the patients' feelings while with the patients. "Using their emotional resources and experiences, physicians connect with patients and support them through myriad distressing situations. Because physicians use themselves as instruments of diagnosis and therapy, personal awareness can help them 'calibrate themselves as instruments,' using themselves more effectively in these capacities" (Novack et al. 1997). A humanistic approach correlates with patients feeling heard, being satisfied, and following medical advice.

What is more, good connections among medical faculty actually improve patient care, education, and research. In hospitals, good interpersonal relationships are linked to better performance by nurses and doctors, and "relationship-centered health care" results in better care and outcomes for the institution (Revans 1996; Suchman 2003; Beach and Inui 2006; Safran et al. 2006; Williams et el. 1998). In this type of care, the doctor explicitly recognizes the patient as a person who lives within a particular social context, not simply a case. The doctor respects the patient's prior experiences and the patient's ideas about what she or he needs (Tresolini 1994).

There is a parallel between disconnection and emotional detachment among medical school faculty and ineffective communication between doctor and patient. If faculty feel disconnected and cannot communicate among themselves, they are less likely to create good relationships with students and patients. Similarly, in a culture where faculty and administrators themselves do not receive consideration and compassion, it is less likely that they will treat students and patients with compassion.

Relationships and Medical Education

Research has also shown that positive relationships are beneficial in education. The eminent psychologist Carl Rogers demonstrated that forming relationships built on trust between teacher and learner is pivotal to facilitate learning (Rogers 1983; Daloz 1999). In middle schools, Bryk and Schneider demonstrated that building trust in a school community, through respectful discourse and nurturing relationships among teachers, parents, and pupils, was the single attribute associated with improved standardized test scores in the children (Bryk and Schneider 2003). Other research has found that trust is required for effective education in a variety of educational settings. This is true in medical education, as in other places of learning.

Teaching may be the hardest and bravest task for medical school faculty. Even though they may be expert in the content of what they teach, many faculty members have received little or no explicit training in how to teach, or in the theories and processes of learning. Medical educators are challenged to prepare trainees to provide high quality, compassionate health care that is responsive to the current and emerging needs of patients as well as to the changing health care system. To do so, graduates must be able to work collaboratively with colleagues and to be competent, self-directed, lifelong learners. To foster these qualities, medical schools need to create a climate of trust in the classroom and among faculty, where the natural desire to learn can be nourished and enhanced (ABIM 1992).

Little direct evidence exists in the literature about the formative experiences of medical faculty and the influence of these experiences on current teaching practices. The study of four medical schools described above which found such high levels of depression among faculty, notes: "Current medical students are being taught by faculty who are increasingly stressed and dispirited"—hardly a positive environment for developing compassion and positive relationships.

As part of the curriculum change process at the medical school in North Carolina, my research team explored medical faculty attitudes, experiences, and values about teaching. We were particularly interested in the extent to which prior experiences might have been formative for faculty members' current teaching behaviors and skills. We reasoned that attempting to understand formative faculty experiences would better enable us to tailor future faculty development interventions to meet faculty needs. When asked about feedback they had received as students, many faculty could only recall feeling unsupported and negatively judged. Most recounted instances of evaluation (judging performance against a gold standard) rather than feedback or coaching designed to improve performance. Humiliation, embarrassment, and strong negative feelings frequently accompanied the evaluations, which were routinely perceived as personal and unfair. Such experiences eroded the trust and potentially positive relationships between teacher and learner. Dr. Cragen's experience was typical:

> I was a third-year medical student, first clerkship, second presentation ever. [I] started presenting a patient. It was in internal medicine so a very complex patient. About ten minutes into the presentation—and being a compulsive third year student I was leaving absolutely nothing out—the attending interrupted and raked me over the coals about not having properly organized the presentation and went on for maybe five minutes doing that—and completely destroyed me as a student at that point. I think I certainly learned a lot from that, I learned to better organize my presentations. Also learned to avoid that particular attending.

The contrast between this person's experience and the type of connection many faculty in our interviews said they sought with their students is striking. Supporting relationship formation in medical schools would surely improve physician education and ameliorate the sometimes negative nature of medical school.

The "Hidden Curriculum"

In exchange for the trust placed in them and the privilege they enjoy, physicians commit to the primacy of patient welfare, making their own needs subservient to those of the patient and to the obligation to provide care for all persons with honesty and integrity. Physicians also must respect patient autonomy. The Charter on Professionalism (ABIM 2002) defines the obligations of medical professionalism as "professional competence, honesty with patients, patient confidentiality, maintaining appropriate relations with patients, improving quality of care, improving access to care, a just distribution of finite resources, scientific knowledge, and maintaining trust by managing conflicts of interest."

The importance of relationships is increasingly being recognized, to the point where new accreditation standards mandate "interpersonal and communication skills and professionalism" for residency training and state that "medical schools (including faculty) must ensure that the learning environment for medical students promotes the development of explicit and appropriate professional attributes in their medical students"

(ACGME n.d.; AAMC 2007). Yet few experts seem to recognize (or address) the fact that the current medical school environment creates significant barriers to developing these professional attributes and humanistic approaches to patients.

A substantial literature describes the informal "hidden curriculum" for medical students, who experience behaviors and attitudes, embodied in the organizational approach and their experiences in medical training, that contrast with the school's stated mission (Snyder 1971; Hafferty and Franks 1994). In effect, students undergo tacit social conditioning and learn certain informal norms and values that are often at odds with humanistic and ethical comportment (Dans 1996; Hundert et al. 1996; Coulehan and Williams 2001; Pololi and Frankel 2001; Pololi et al. 2001; Hojat et al. 2004). For example, a 1994 study found that 98 percent of medical students observed physicians referring to patients in a derogatory way; the students reported that they felt obliged to "fit in" with this behavior (Feudtner and Christakis 1994).

With this background, over the four years of medical school, medical students tend to lose the humanistic and altruistic attitudes they originally brought to their training (Coombs 1978; McKegney 1989; Crandall et al. 1993; Hundert et al. 1996; Coulehan and Williams 2001; Hojat et al. 2004; Woloschuk et al. 2004; Dyrbye et al. 2005). Studies have shown that medical students become less empathic as they progress though medical school (Hojat et al. 2004). They learn that "affective neutrality," or suppressing their feelings for patients and their suffering, is a goal to strive for (Pololi and Frankel 2001; Pololi et al. 2001). It is perhaps not coincidental that recent studies in a consortium of seven medical schools showed that 49 percent of medical students demonstrate signs of burnout and 11 percent reported suicidal ideation during the first two years of medical school as well as very high levels of psychological stress (Dyrbye et al. 2009).

Not surprisingly, the "hidden curriculum" has been linked to unprofessional and unethical behavior among medical students (Crandall et al. 1993). This "progressive decline of moral reasoning during undergraduate medical school training" (Self et al. 1989; Dans 1996; Rennie and Rudland 2003; Woloshuk et al. 2004), may also contribute to future unprofessional behaviors. Sonia Crandall found that medical students "became less favorably inclined to caring for the medically indigent over the four years of medical school"—although interestingly, this was not the case with female students (Crandall et al. 1993). Instead of learning to be humanistic, socially responsible, and compassionate, and receiving training that nurtures their self-awareness and emotional development, medical students learn that they will be rewarded for individual achievement, self-promotion, and being lead author on publications, rather than collaborative efforts (Cuff and Vanselow 2004). Unethical behaviors observed in students included academic dishonesty or cheating, as well as "dishonesty in patient care activities, such as recording tasks not performed, reporting findings elicited by others, and lying about ordering a test, often motivated by fear and a desire to appear knowledgeable" (Dyrbye et al. 2005).

In this way medical school culture erects barriers to learning and team building as well as to compassionate care (Kassebaum and Cutler 1998). The different responses among female medical students reported by Crandall align with our own findings that female faculty held onto their own values and experienced greater discomfort than did men over the disjuncture between these values and those of the institution (see Chapter 5).

A "Latent Curriculum" Among Medical Faculty

Our interviews describe a "latent curriculum," consisting of expectations and consequent conditioning among medical school faculty that is similar to the "hidden curriculum" for medical students. Through these expectations, faculty learn that the actions that are rewarded are not always those the institution holds up officially as its ideals. For example, Dr. Door discovered that her hospital would provide compassionate care only to those who could afford it—not to all:

> I want to take care of patients and I found that some of my poorer patients would come to see me and [would hear] "Your insurance has lapsed or your Medicaid" or this or that and "We can't see you now." I felt that the administration people were getting in the way of what I wanted to do because they have another agenda . . . so I couldn't see my patients.

She eventually left academic medicine.

What makes this a truly critical issue is that medical faculty are models for their students, so that the source of the "hidden curriculum" of a medical school is the "latent curriculum" experienced by its faculty. This tacit conditioning is well illustrated by a story told to me by a female medical student:

> I had looked forward to my first clinical experience in medicine. I had even enjoyed the first two years of medical school because I saw that a good part of what I was learning would be helpful in understanding and helping patients. I viewed a physician as a professional who was part of a community and provided holistic care for his or her patients. I looked forward to learning the practice of medicine from talented, wise, caring mentors. I was therefore taken aback to learn on my first rotation in a prestigious hospital that there were 'interesting" patients and "not-interesting" patients. I was shocked to be sent to do a paracentesis on a poor alcoholic patient without supervision. I was silenced from expressing my learning needs on rounds, where the point seemed to be to demonstrate what you knew rather than reveal anything you didn't. Primary care physicians were frequently spoken of in disparaging terms. And we were on for thirty-six hours and off for twelve hours, which was personally grueling. Luckily this was juxtaposed with a fourth year externship working with a resident who was supportive, caring, and "learner-centered," although I had not heard of the term then.

The "latent curriculum" operates among research scientists as well. A culture that trains scientists to compete and considers expressing emotions as a form of weakness, seriously impedes interdisciplinary and collaborative work in the biomedical sciences. People wedded to competitive individualism will not be effective collaborators. This too is now a critical issue, because science is changing, and scientific advances require research across disciplines. For example, teams of researchers that include practicing physicians as well as laboratory scientists are more likely to produce advances in scientific knowledge that can be rapidly translated and applied to improved patient care. Good relationships among colleagues facilitate the success of interdisciplinary clinical teams and multidisciplinary research collaborations.

For this reason, the NIH has recommended interdisciplinary collaboration as a priority for scientific discovery and translation of new knowledge to clinical outcomes (NIH 2008). In 2004, Elias Zerhouni, the Director of NIH at the time, established a new Roadmap for Medical Research "to address roadblocks to research and to transform the way biomedical research is conducted." This innovative and "crosscutting" research program specifically called for a "change in the academic culture to foster collaboration."

Collaboration involves developing relationships, learning to understand other people's perspectives, and communicating effectively; in the long term, it also requires some enjoyment of working with other team members. Although team members' ideas and expertise are essential, their emotions are also important, since these affect their own work and that of the group. The challenge, then, is to revise the "latent curriculum" so as to support faculty ability to collaborate. At the same time, such change would bring great improvements in the culture of the medical school in general.

Supportive personal connections among faculty can enhance the experience of working in an academic medical center and facilitate the work of caring for patients, teaching physicians in training, carrying out leadership and management responsibilities, and conducting biomedical and behavioral research.

Parts of this chapter have been published as: Pololi L, Conrad P, Knight S, Carr P. A study of the relational aspects of the culture of academic medicine. Acad Med. 2009;84:106–14.

REFERENCES

ABIM Foundation; ACP-ASIM Foundation; European Federation of Internal Medicine. Medical professionalism in the new millennium. A physician charter. Ann Intern Med. 2002;136:243–246.

Accreditation Council on Graduate Medical Education (ACGME). Available at: http://www.acgme.org/acWebsite/home/home.asp.

American Board of Internal Medicine. Guide to awareness and evaluation of humanistic qualities in the internist. Philadelphia: ABIM; 1992.

Association of American Medical Colleges. 2007 LCME Standard MS-31-A. Available at: http://www.lcme.org/standard.htm.

Beach MC, Inui TS, Network R-C-CR. Relationship-centered care: a constructive reframing. J Gen Intern Med. 2006;21:S3–8.

Bryk AS, Schneider BL. Trust in schools: a core resource for school reform. Educ Leadership. 2003;60:40.

Burns JM. Leadership. New York: Harper & Row; 1978.

Coombs RH. Mastering medicine: Professional socialization in medical school. New York: Free Press; 1978.

Coulehan J, Williams JD. Vanquishing virtue: the impact of medical education. Acad Med. 2001;76:598–605.

Crandall SJ, Volk RJ, Loemker V. Medical students' attitudes toward providing care for the underserved: are we training socially responsible physicians? JAMA. 1993;269:2519–23.

Cuff PA, Vanselow NA. Improving medical education: Enhancing the behavioral and social science content of medical school curricula [IOM report]. Washington, DC: The National Academies Press; 2004.

Daloz L. Guiding the journey of adult learners. San Francisco: Jossey-Bass; 1999.

Dans PE. Self-reported cheating by students at one medical school. Acad Med. 1996;71(1):S70–2.

Dyrbye LN, Thomas MR, Massie FS, Power DV, Eacker A, Harper W, Durning S, Moutier C, Szydlo DW, Novotny PJ, Sloan JA, Shanafelt TD. Burnout and suicidal ideation among U.S. medical students. Ann Intern Med. 2009;149: 334–41.

Dyrbye LN, Thomas MR, Shanafelt TD. Medical student distress: causes, consequences, and proposed solutions. Mayo Clin Proc. 2005;80(12):1613–22.

Feudtner C, Christakis CA. Do clinical clerks suffer ethical erosion? Students' perceptions of their clinical environment and personal development. Acad Med. 1994;69:670–9.

Fugelli P. Trust in general practice: The James Mackenzie Lecture, 2000. Br J Gen Pract. 2001;51:575–9.

Hafferty FW, Franks R. The hidden curriculum, ethics teaching and the structure of medical education. Acad Med. 1994;69:861–71.

Hartling L, Sparks E. Relational cultural practice: working in a nonrelational world. Work in progress no. 97. Wellesley, MA: Stone Center, Wellesley College; 2002.

Hauck FR, Zyzanski SJ, Alemagno SA, Medalie JH. Patient perceptions of humanism in physicians: effects on positive health behaviors. Family Med. 1990; 22(6):447–52.

Hojat M, Mangione S, Nasca TJ, Rattner S, Erdmann JB, Gonnella JS, Magee M. An empirical study of decline in empathy in medical school. Medical Education. 2004;38:934–41.

Hundert EM, Hafferty FW, Christakis DA. Characteristics of the informal curriculum and trainees' ethical choices. Acad Med. 1996;71:624–33.

Kassebaum DG, Cutler ER. On the culture of student abuse in medical school. Acad Med. 1998;73(11):1149–58.

Luhmann N. Trust and power. New York: John Wiley & Sons; 1979.

Martinson BC, Anderson MS, de Vries R. Scientists behaving badly. Nature. 2005;435:737–8.

Maslach C. Burnout: the cost of caring. Englewood Cliffs, NJ: Prentice-Hall; 1982.

McKegney CP. Medical education: A neglectful and abusive family system. Family Med. 1989;21(6):452–7.

McMurray JE, Linzer M, Konrad T, Douglas J, Shugerman R, Nelson KJ. The work lives of women physicians: results from the physician work life study. J Gen Intern Med. 2000;15:372–80.

National Institutes of Health. http://nihroadmap.nih.gov/interdisciplinary/explora torycenters/. Reviewed January 23, 2008.

Novack DH, Suchman AL, Clark W, Epstein RM, Najberg E, Kaplan C. Calibrating the physician: personal awareness and effective patient care. JAMA. 1997; 278(6):502.

Pololi L, Frankel RM. Small group teaching emphasizing reflection can positively influence medical students' values. Acad Med. 2001;76:1172–3.

Pololi L, Frankel RM, Clay M, Jobe AC. One year's experience with a program to facilitate personal and professional development in medical students using reflection groups. Educ Health. 2001;14:36–9.

Rennie SC, Rudland JR. Differences in medical students' attitudes to academic misconduct and reported behavior across the years—a questionnaire study. J Med Ethics. 2003;29:97–102.

Revans RW. The hospital as a human system. Bull NY Acad Med. 1996;73: 418–29.

Rogers C. The interpersonal relationship in the facilitation of learning. Freedom to learn for the 80's. Columbus, OH: Bell & Howell Co; 1983:119–34.

Safran DG, Miller W, Beckman HB. Organizational dimensions of relationship-centered care: theory, evidence and practice. J Gen Intern Med. 2006;21:S9–15.

Schindler BA, Novack DH, Cohen DG, Yager J, Wang D, Shaheen NJ, Guze P, Wilkerson L, Drossman DA. The impact of the changing health care environment on the health and well-being of faculty at four medical schools. Acad Med. 2006;81:27–34.

Self DJ, Wolinsky FD, Baldwin DC. The effect of teaching medical ethics on medical students' moral reasoning. Acad Med. 1989;64:755–9.

Seligman AB. The problem of trust. Princeton, NJ: Princeton University Press; 1997.

Shanafelt T, Sloan J, Haberman T. The well-being of physicians. Am J Med. 2003;114:513–9.

Shanafelt TD, West CP, Sloan JA, Novotny PJ, Poland GA, Menaker R, Rummans TA, Dyrbe LN. Career fit and burnout among academic faculty. Arch Intern Med. 2009;168:990–5.

Snyder BR. The hidden curriculum. New York: Alfred A. Knopf; 1971.

Spickard A, Gabbe SG, Christensen J. Mid-career burnout in generalist and specialist physicians. JAMA. 2002;288:1447–50.

Suchman AL. Relationship-centered administration. In: Quill TE, Frankel RM, McDaniel SH, eds. The biopsychosocial approach: past, present, future. Rochester, NY: University of Rochester Press; 2003.

Suchman AL, Botelho RJ, Hinton-Walker P, eds. Partnerships in healthcare: transforming relational process. Rochester, NY: University of Rochester Press; 1998.

Tresolini CP, The Pew Fetzer Task Force on Psychosocial Education. Health professions education and relationship-centered care: report of the Pew-Fetzer Task Force on Advancing Psychosocial Education. San Francisco: Pew Health Commission; 1994, 1–76.

Woloschuk W, Harasym PH, Temple W. Attitude change during medical school: a cohort study. Med Educ. 2004;38:522–34.

chapter 5

Values and Trust in Academic Medicine

> Schools are the sanctuaries of our personal and civic values and incubators of intellect and integrity. The values that mark our community are the values most likely to be learned by our students. —E. Grady Bogue (2002)

As the two preceding chapters have shown, medical faculty value deeply their work in teaching, research, and caring for patients. In the late 1990s, I conducted an assessment to determine what faculty required in order to keep learning and to sustain their professional vitality. I needed that information in order to design for them the professional development program mentioned previously. I also asked key leaders and administrators a related question: What characteristics or attributes does a faculty member need to help the medical school achieve its goals? The answers from these two groups regarding faculty needs were very different (Pololi 2003).

Faculty listed their three top needs as "maintaining my academic vitality," "retaining my own values," and "balancing personal and professional demands." "Time management" was rated fourth, and they identified "finding meaning in my work" as their fifth priority. Senior administrators, by contrast, prioritized as faculty needs "time management," "managerial and executive skills," and "an attitude that has an institutional edge," as well as "flexibility," "teamwork," "collaborative skills," "advocacy for students," and "the ability to think globally beyond a department." This variance between the importance of values and vitality on the personal level, on the one hand, and the institutional perspective of how best to serve the organization's needs, on the other, suggests that administrators were largely unaware of the faculty's need for professional support and renewal in order for them to be effective and contribute their best to the institution.

Building on this earlier work, our research interviews for the C - Change project sought to understand what faculty valued most in their work. What aspects of it mattered most to them and what motivated them to go on doing this work in the face of (in many cases) considerable difficulties and challenges? Based on their responses, we identified four dimensions that were most important to faculty:

> *The social mission to provide health care to all.* Faculty expressed a deep-seated belief that physicians, medical schools, and the health care system overall had a responsibility to support this mission, which faculty saw as a basic tenet of the profession. It meant, in particular, not being obliged to select which patients to care for.
>
> *The responsibility to advance medical knowledge.* Faculty saw this not only as a societal value but also expressed real personal excitement at the wonderment of science.
>
> *The mission of teaching future physicians.* Faculty saw educating young people as another important responsibility that was also personally gratifying.
>
> A *sense of professional ethics,* the core of which was putting the patient first.

We also asked each faculty member what they perceived their institution to value and whether their own professional values were aligned or in conflict with what the institution considered important. In response, many faculty members described behaviors and actions leading them to conclude that their medical school did not place the same value on education or the social mission of clinical care, and that it sometimes seemed to value research more for the grant money it brought in than for the intrinsic importance of scientific outcomes. Faculty were also disturbed by occasional perceived unethical behavior on the part of some administrators or other faculty members. Thus, many on the faculty felt a conflict between their personal values and the behaviors and expectations of the institutions where they worked.

I believe this values conflict is a key issue. People work at their optimum level when what they do aligns with their own values. If we want medical faculty to be able to function at their best, we need to ensure that the institutions where they work support those values. And if the institutions do not, it is essential to be aware of this disconnect, since it has a significant effect on the faculty's ability to be fully engaged in their work.

Our research shows that, in fact, the existing academic medical system does not always allow faculty to function in accordance with their values and ideals. The results, which are similar to the earlier needs assessment, suggest that medical school leaders are often unaware that this is a problem for their faculty. Yet, these leaders must fully understand this problem where it exists if their schools are to draw on their faculty's full potential and benefit from all the contributions the faculty are capable of.

At the same time, it must be recognized that many academic medical centers are undergoing a financial crisis, one effect of which is to put pressure on faculty to generate increased revenue by seeing additional patients with less time allocated to each clinical encounter. Securing research funding has also become increasingly competitive. As a result, not only are faculty left with less time, energy, or reward for teaching or research; they also find themselves unable to give patients the kind of quality care they believe it is their duty to deliver. This problem raises the question: How can we support faculty and help them attain professional fulfillment within these budgetary constraints?

Social Mission

In the interviews, women faculty often told us that they remained in academic medicine rather than go into private practice in order to better fulfill the social mission of medicine. Part of their motivation was a need to look after "the community" and vulnerable populations. Many academic medical centers, especially those in large urban areas, are located in neighborhoods housing large groups of underserved people, especially the poor, minority groups, and recent immigrants. For faculty members, caring for these vulnerable groups, who are less able to access health care or who do not often receive the same quality of care as more privileged or educated people, was an important professional responsibility. They felt they could fulfill this social mission in a medical school hospital, whereas in private practice this would be less likely or impossible.

> Dr. Cole: My values. . . . [are] to provide health care, education for the community at large and for the underserved community, and to pay particular attention to diversity in people and thinking.

Dr. Ireland: I will stay here forever probably, because I do feel a very high social responsibility to care for people who really have no choice.

Dr. Wall, an obstetrician: Academic medicine aligns very closely with what I think is correct and ethical, in the sense that I can provide care to patients, and I never have to ask anybody whether they have insurance or not. And I don't ever have to ask anybody if they can pay. If you come to the hospital and you're sick, I'm going to take care of you. And that's the ideal way to practice medicine, in my opinion. But I also recognize that when you're in private practice, you've got to make a living and you can't do that.

Dr. Francesco, an internist: Probably, my most basic value is social justice. What has often motivated me has been standing up for the underdog, whether that was the learner, or the patient, or the quieter person, or the woman, or the underrepresented minority. I tend to become more courageous when I perceive an underdog of some sort. I think that has informed a lot of my work. And in fact, I think I don't really like overdogs. If there's an opposite of an underdog, it's an overdog. I have only just thought of that word.

Interviewer: "Top dog?"

Dr. Francesco: "Top dog." Right—there's something about top dogs that irritates me a bit.

In Chapter 3 we saw Dr. Francesco describing "the enormous trust that a patient can place in a physician and really the privilege the physician has of holding that trust." To her, this was a value that "I held very dear and I felt really important for the practice of medicine, or for a medical school to uphold."

Betrayal of the Public Trust

In stark contrast to these expressions of altruism was the conviction that academic medicine had lost its social mission and was betraying its public trust. Many physicians felt very stressed by the requirement to increase the number of patients seen each day, with less time allocated for each; they were disheartened by the consequent reduction in the attention and care they could provide to individual patients. They saw this as adversely affecting patient care and also as undermining the social mission of the medical center.

Lack of Support for Excellence in Patient Care

Numerous faculty commented, often in heated or ironic tones, on the lack of support for clinical care (i.e., taking care of patients). They thought their institution did not place a very high priority on clinical excellence and did not provide adequate funding to achieve it. They described the academic medical center as taking an entrepreneurial approach. Dr. Jerry explained that the medical center was not willing to hire additional support staff because it could not directly bill the patient (or insurance company) for the time spent by support staff caring for the patient, whereas it could charge much more for physician time and services.

> Dr. Jerry: Oh, it's all money. Anybody that says otherwise doesn't understand the workings of academics. There's great lip service about the academic mission and patient care comes first. I wish that were true. If it were, I would feel very differently about these places. But it's not. It's how many [patients] you can do in clinic: "You're seeing 3.4 people per room; you should be seeing 3.6 people per room." It's all about money and that's the bottom line. They will not give you support because they don't want to spend any more money on the support staff: "They don't generate their own salaries."

> Dr. Schmidt: I feel that I'm not able to do enough for my patients, given some of the lack of resources we have. And that is frustrating.

Another faculty member noted that while the public expects to receive highly expert care in an academic medical center from super-specialists, the faculty whom the institution most values and tries to recruit are more likely to excel at basic research and may be less skilled in clinical care.

> Dr. Alford: I think everybody has to reexamine what it is to be in academic medicine—and it really came to light for me about a year ago,

when I was on a search committee for a division chief in another department. We were there in a group interviewing, and every single candidate that came in talked about how they needed to protect their faculty from clinical work. Patients come here expecting the most experienced and the most savvy clinicians because it's a big university academic medical center. Yet there are faculty members here who perform way less or see way fewer patients than the private guy down the street. So there's a falsehood of how people here perceive themselves and how the public sees it. People look at a place like this and say "Well, I'm certainly going to go there if I have something really serious." Yet you're going to see people who practice the least amount of medicine. In this day and age, patients are more complex, you have more data to deal with, and there have been several studies to show that those who practice certain things the most are the best at it. It really is a sheer number-driven thing. If you do the most, you are the best in terms of outcome and complications.

At the same time, although clinicians' patient-care-related activities brought in money that often helped to keep the research enterprise going, the clinicians felt they were not valued as much as researchers. Whereas clinical work generated sizable income, research funding garnered more prestige.

Dr. McGuire: Publications and being invited to speak at other institutions, getting a lot of grants, that is valued, higher than patient care. If you were to ask somebody, who is most accomplished—those people are not necessarily the most adept at patient care, which I find interesting.

Another faculty member, Dr. Alexis, confirmed:

You hear the talk through the halls and then you can tell what the culture is, and even though they say clinicians are the life blood of the institution, the researchers are perceived to be more valuable. Now mind you, I know they have stress because they're being told: "You only have a million dollar grant, you need more grant funding and if you lose this grant, you're out of here." So they have their problems and I have mine.

Many teaching hospitals operate in the red, so they need to bring in as much clinical income as possible. But as these quotes indicate, seeing too many patients did not always equate with providing high-quality care. As Dr. Scarlet put it, her administration was willing to make decisions for financial benefit that lost sight of the very reason for the existence of the organization: to care for patients. She seemed better able than most to articulate her values and apply them to her everyday decisions and actions, and she had the courage to raise this issue with other doctors and with administrators.

> Dr. Scarlet: I do some things arbitrarily at times, like the next person, but insofar as I am able, I try to apply my values to everything. In my discussions with the dean, he is always talking about "no money—no mission," and I understand what he is saying: if we can't keep the doors open financially, then we won't take care of any sick folks; we won't train any medical students. But my point to him was that if we lose sight of what we are here for, we have no reason to keep our doors open. I think the focus is too much on the bottom line, to the point where we talk about giving up what makes us physicians in the first place. I've been on the board for the financial aspects of a university physicians' group, and there was a discussion one day about whether we should have crash carts, because if we do it increases our liability, etc. Some comments were made that we should just eliminate the crash carts and call 911 if somebody collapses in our clinic, and I said, "Wait a minute, this is ridiculous, are we physicians or are we not, what are we here for? What are we doing?"

Another internist, Dr. Winter, who had developed a hospice program to care for dying patients, described meeting with a senior administrator in her hospital system. The administrator said, "How can we make money if the patients are just coming to die here. . . . We have to make more money while we are doing the hospice care." She told me that she cried after the meeting, feeling that she had an ethical responsibility to care for dying patients, regardless of how little income this hospice practice brought in. Unwilling to alter her practice with these patients to generate more clinical charges, Dr. Winter concluded that this institution was "not where I belonged." She left and continues her work outside academic medicine.

Dr. Francesco mused on the contradiction between the current organization of academic medicine and the goal of creating trusting relationships with patients. She did not think the military-type hierarchical organization of the academic medical center, which demanded unquestioning obedience from the powerless, was well suited to carry out the medical mission of serving the patient. Dr. Francesco described it thus:

> There's this whole hierarchical structure where one tells the other what to do, and the person passes it down the line, until you get to the lowest rungs of the ladder. So it's like a military set up, which is somehow antithetical to the practice of medicine—where the final outcome is that you are trying to form this trusting relationship between the physician and the patient, so the physician can be responsive and helpful regarding the patient's suffering. And of course there is a lot of power in that relationship too, the physician has enormous power, and the patient has very little power, and most patients feel that power differential. On the other hand, the primacy of the patient and the whole professional ethic is that the physician will hold in trust the patient's well-being. And never compromise that.

Lack of Commitment to the Community

Many medical faculty recognized that even though part of their school's avowed mission was service to the local community, this commitment was not fulfilled in practice. We heard comments such as, "academic medicine is hypocritical." Some faculty felt bitterly disappointed by what they saw as a lack of social purpose and responsibility in academic medicine.

> Dr. Allen: There's no leadership; there's no vision; there's no intelligence; there's no proud foot forward; there's no cohesiveness about where the country needs to go; there's no sense of purpose. It's just all churning water. So while we have this emerging technology and the ability to treat patients, we have no sense of social purpose or social policy.

We heard much disdain for the current state of the nation's health care system as well as for what interviewees considered an inappropriately corporate culture in their medical school.

> Dr. Alpert: I'm somewhat cynical at this point because the whole health care system is broken. And so my values in serving the community and having health care for everybody are not fostered in the university setting or in most university settings. I think that our society should support ed-

ucation in a different way. Universities are looking much more like corporations than they used to. I hear the same kind of business-speak at the university as I heard in the private, for-profit company I worked for. In fact, there are fewer differences than ever before, so I think it's become a business. And I don't think that's where education should be, and I also don't think that's where health care should be.

Thus, many of these interviewees raised the question of whether academic medicine is betraying the public trust and failing to live up to its professed social mission.

Intellectual Mission

Interviewees prized their role as scientific researchers and their intellectual freedom, both of which they saw as integral to their role as faculty. As we saw in Chapter 3, they loved the excitement of scientific inquiry and took great satisfaction in seeing their discoveries translated into clinical applications and rewarded with publication. Dr. Ireland, a physician scientist, and Dr. Haitham, a researcher, both exemplify these feelings.

> Dr. Ireland: I had my own lab, . . . there was an unbelievably driving passion to answer questions in a way that would add to the information that will make children's lives better. I saw that for me, clinical care was never going to be enough. I needed to take my intellect and drive it as far as I could. That meant getting support doing experiments in the laboratory, presenting my results and getting published . . . the purpose of getting published was to get the information out. What kept me in academics when things have not been so good over the years was the richness of asking, answering questions and then being able to share that with other people.

> Dr. Haitham: Making a difference in people's lives at the end of the day means an incredible amount to me, and I've got two large studies going at the moment testing new interventions. If one of them really turns out to be effective, there's no better feeling in the world.

Others, like Dr. Sanders, a senior physician researcher, spoke of science serving the social mission. She was studying how certain types of illness are manifested and treated differently in different racial groups:

Dr. Sanders: My research also opened the door to the whole question of how we use race in medicine. So there was a social part and there's a science part, and I guess I would have to say that that's probably been the highest point.

The Influence of Money on Research

Traditionally, a specified portion of a faculty member's salary was understood to cover time spent on research. The goal was to get a grant to cover that part of the salary, but even if that person's grant applications did not always bring in funding, the research time was supported. Now, however, with this type of funded research position shrinking, our interviewees perceived that the ability to bring in grant money was valued more than the quality of someone's work or the knowledge gained.

Dr. Brown described how "the push for the clinical dollar" squeezed out the time that could be devoted to "traditional scholarly work," meaning not only research that followed a rigorous scientific process but also publishing and presenting results at scientific meetings:

> The push for the clinical dollar is greater than ever. And how one can resolve that with the need to do scholarly work—all I can say is, it happens with great difficulty. More and more, I think people are having to decide that even though they join an academic institution, they will be among the group that is not expected to do what has been traditional scholarly work. And that is very sad because I don't know what academic institutions are going to turn into.

Another woman noted how this focus on money affected medical advances:

> Dr. Flower: A lot of things are tied to money, so I think that research or publications or important advancements are sometimes not developed because they're not funded.

Often, even when someone received funding for the research itself, she had to write about it on her own time. Many of our interviewees complained that they did not have the time to publish, yet without publishing they could not get promotions, recognition, or more funding. We heard comments like, "I have a pile of data on my desk, and I write about it at 3 a.m."

Dr. Barkman noted, "Very few of us get into a permanent position in academia with a guaranteed salary, and that is shrinking." She was alluding to the fact that fewer academic physicians are getting tenure. An individual in a nontenured job might have a one-year or three-year contract allowing a percentage of her time to pursue research. However, she would be aware that her real worth to the institution was based on the clinical income she brought in and that her employment could be reevaluated if she did not bring in the expected amount.

Tenure decisions too can be influenced by the amount of external research funding a faculty member brings in. In addition to the award amount, which goes to the investigator to cover salaries, supplies, and other direct expenses, the NIH give the university at least 50 percent above that amount in additional funding to cover overhead expenses. Dr. Barkman referred to the value to the university of grant money from the NIH: "If you have shown that you can publish as well as have federal money which comes with close to 50 percent overhead, you're set. If you only have publications and no track record of funding outside the university, you will not get tenure."

At least in part because of these disincentives, there are insufficient numbers of physician-scientists in our medical schools, which have not yet found ways to adequately support the time needed for faculty to conduct research.

Perhaps as a consequence of this focus on money, interviewees reported occasional disturbing incidents of unethical behavior. Dr. Haitham, for example, explained that because such behavior was often condoned by those in power, she had to go along with it in order to continue doing her work.

> About a year into being here, I realized that though I just wanted to be
> a bench scientist, the greed [pervasive in the environment] doesn't allow
> you to simply be a good worker and be happy, because somebody controls
> your life. And when people who control your life are not very good, they
> are not using their integrity or scruples, you are confronted with being
> controlled by someone like that. It was just a very sudden realization and

> I said, ah, I better change my plans, I better become independent. And I
> just walked out and said to my boss, "I'm leaving; I got a job elsewhere."

Other faculty described discomfort over poor compliance with federally
mandated rules safeguarding people involved as research subjects. An
example might be a clinical study that entails strict rules about informed
consent. The investigator must attest to having fully explained the experiment to patients so they understand the risks and can make a well-
informed decision about whether to participate. Either because of conve-
nience or expedience, an investigator might not fully explain the risk, and
if patients do not read all the documents or understand them well, they
may not in fact understand these risks. Yet the investigator still affirms
having obtained informed consent from all study participants. Dr. Haitham explained that if in order to maintain her integrity she refused to
behave in a similar unethical way, she could be fired or at the least would
be unable to do her research.

Dr. Door, another researcher, questioned the influence of money on her
own behavior—whether research interests were taking priority over patient well being. She was studying the effectiveness of vaccines and tried to
clarify for herself whether she was behaving professionally and ethically.

> I did a couple of vaccine studies, and now I've got to get patients to go
> along with taking this particular new vaccine that we're trialing, and it's
> a baby, and you say to yourself, "well, am I doing something wrong
> here?". . . . You tell the patient [parent] about your study and inform
> [her/him] what tests [she/he] will have based on receiving this specific
> study medicine. And you say to yourself, "Are you doing something be-
> cause of the money?" For every patient you get, $250 goes to the depart-
> ment. You're offering the patient some sort of reward too, and that's
> what's swaying the patient who has no money, versus somebody who
> has. So on that level, maybe I compromise my values a little bit, but I
> always think to myself, "Is this a good study? Is this something that ul-
> timately is going to help all children?" And then in my head I said "yes,"
> because the vaccines that were coming out were good, and I don't think
> I compromised myself on that level. But I'd have to say it feels funny
> when you're trying to convince somebody to do something that maybe
> you wouldn't as a mother want for your own kid.

Much literature addresses the conflict between commercialism and professional values in medicine. Working relationships between academic medical centers and industry have grown to create powerful financial conflicts of interest. As a result, institutions and individual faculty feel pressure to compromise their traditional academic values. As Jordan Cohen, former president of the AAMC, said: "The ability to benefit optimally from growing relationships with industry is heavily dependent on remaining true to fundamental academic values, including the safety of human subjects research, the integrity of the scientific process, and the free exchange of research results" (Cohen and Siegel 2005).

Teaching

Teaching is awarded less prestige than funded research or clinical work, even when a faculty member is an outstanding educator. Yet, although medical faculty generally receive little or no training in teaching, they know it is an essential mission of academic medicine and an important part of their work responsibilities. Many derive substantial gratification and stimulation from teaching students and also from other scholarly activities, such as the study of medical education. For some, teaching medical students and residents, together with undertaking curriculum reform or educational innovation, are the very reasons they chose a career in academic medicine instead of private practice.

> Dr. Grant: Getting into academic medicine has fulfilled a lot of those desires, because you teach. Part of it is teaching others how to become a scientist or a physician, and you're perpetuating this wonderful field.

> Dr. Goldsmith: And feeling good about teaching, educating, teaching the next generation of surgeons.

> Dr. Ireland: It is extremely rewarding to me to try and explain something to another person, residents, fellows . . . that type of thing. It's such a rich environment.

Some people pointed out the importance of having students learn the practice of medicine outside the acute care hospital, since this is where most health care delivery takes place. One described her gratification at seeing how much her students benefited from teaching by community physicians:

> Dr. Conevarez: They're the real teachers in my mind. That's the more real part of learning. The community physicians loved teaching students, and the students loved it. It was a great experience for the students, for the physicians, and personally satisfying to me because that was my job, helping change the university. So that's what I mean by the unreal world—getting students outside the disparaging, know-it-all, self-serving faculty (that's the stereotype), to the cooperative, wonderful, charming, caring physician out in the community.

Teaching Compromised

Medical education follows an apprenticeship model in which most teaching involves students accompanying physicians as they see patients. However, the financial pressure to see more patients can affect this teaching, as it does patient care. Since the physician has often only ten minutes to see each patient during clinic or ward rounds, she has no time to provide detailed explanations and discuss patients with students, who are left to pick up whatever they can from observation only. Many faculty complained that they did not have enough time to teach their students and residents well and thought that the quality of the education offered to students was compromised. Dr. Venetia, a nationally recognized medical educator, further analyzed the negative consequences of the focus on generating income:

> One of the reasons the weak leadership of the educational programs has been allowed to continue is a fear that strong leadership would clash with the need to focus on clinical productivity . . . it would take resources away from the clinical enterprise. I think it is to their advantage to have weak leadership of the educational enterprise. Otherwise, there might be demand that would be difficult or impossible to meet, and that would be a difficult thing to wrestle with, being that they are a school located in a university.

As one person put it, "We were clinical educators, but actually, as far as we could tell, the education part received pretty much lip service from our chair and the associate chair." Another faculty member regretted that educators were not recognized or rewarded for their teaching despite their dedication to this mission.

> Dr. Schmidt: I run the resident clinic. We're not rewarded by the Medical School at all. A few people each year might be recognized, but for the ongoing day-to-day grind, we're not recognized by the medical school for our efforts . . . We basically provide free labor, you might call it, for the school . . . people stay because they feel a dedication to education . . .

Dr. Anderson believed that although in the past she had successfully integrated patient care with teaching, time and financial pressures no longer allowed her to carry out these two roles simultaneously and according to her high standards.

> Dr. Anderson: I think I've been able to carve out a niche for myself where my personal values are very consistent with what I do, in the subjects I teach, in the way that I supervise the students, the way that I work with the residents, and the way that I treat my patients. I think that the increasing pressure to be more clinically productive is starting to come into conflict with those values and perhaps it is one reason why I am leaving.

Dr. Venetia explained that her medical school administration didn't dare say that education was unimportant, since a quality educational program was required to maintain the school's accreditation. Nevertheless, she said, the institution did not value, treat well, or adequately recognize faculty who did this essential work and did it well. She felt that disregard for her own work prevented her from feeling a sense of belonging, and she, too, left academic medicine. "What I thought was important, was no longer what the institution thought was important," she remarked.

> Dr. Venetia: One particular low point was when . . . I felt that my work was no longer valued. On the other hand it was clear that it was needed. In particular, I had been pushing for an overall plan for the medical school curriculum. This is required now by accreditation standards: What's the overall goal? What's our mission as a school? How does that translate into educational programs? And how does it help guide educational programs and frame them? Grudgingly, I was told, "Ok, go ahead

and develop something and write it up." And so I did, and all the time people would say, "We don't need to do this." [Eventually] it became clear that it was absolutely needed, but what I had written was essentially taken over, my name was taken off it, and my superior's name was put on it and presented all over the school—as this other person's work—with no acknowledgment at all that it was my work, something that was important to me. I was very clearly and completely marginalized, and that was distressing—because I was getting very mixed messages. One message was "Oh, this is very important"; the other message was "Oh, but you're not. Thank you very much; we need this but we don't need you." It's a very strange message to be receiving.

Another highly regarded physician educator, Dr. Silverman, agreed that medical schools become responsive to education needs only in response to pressure from external accrediting bodies. She referred to recent mandates issued by the Accreditation Council on Graduate Medical Education (ACGME), which oversees the quality of residency training programs. When she made curriculum suggestions ten years earlier, her supervisors had laughed at her. But then her ideas eventually became accreditation criteria, and the administration discovered that it had to implement them.

> Dr. Silverman: So right now, everybody's smiling and everybody's happy and my values and the institution's values are just starting to line up and I'm getting to contribute in a way that people respect and I enjoy. But I'm not sure [small laugh] if that's just trends or if this is a change that's permanent.

> Interviewer: Are you saying that your institution's values happen to be aligned with yours now, but only because they're [sic] reacting to the external mandates from ACGME?

> Dr. Silverman: Oh, totally. There's no question in my mind about that. It's not that I feel insecure about myself. I do recognize the importance of the work I've been doing. But I just have no reason to believe that they would suddenly see the light—certainly not here, because ten years ago, everybody was smiling [laughing] at this . . . the same people, you know.

And all of a sudden [they changed their mind], and I don't think that they suddenly discovered that they were wrong.

Ethical Lapses

Chapter 4 described an erosion of trust resulting partly from breaches of academic integrity. A troubling finding in our research data was that numerous interviewees, besides Dr. Tonder and Dr. Haitham, described experiences of unethical and dishonest behavior that they felt were tolerated by the institutional leaders. These included dishonest practices in conducting research, stealing ideas, lying about accomplishments to gain advancement, and lapses in financial integrity. Our interviewees' accounts agree with the published study (Martinson et al. 2005) that found startlingly high levels of unethical conduct among NIH-funded scientists, also described in Chapter 4.

Many interviewees said that honesty was important to them. One woman put it bluntly:

> Dr. Francesco: Well, I guess I'm very taken by truthfulness. I'm really not willing to compromise at all in terms of truthfulness. I think I'm less willing to compromise in terms of truthfulness than most people are. I have recognized this. Such that it may be a failing. [laughs]

She speculated that the prevalence of dishonesty was a result of the prevailing environment.

> Dr. Francesco: I really believe in the intrinsic goodness of people and that most people are well intentioned and trying to do their best, and they end up doing things that aren't so great just because of their experiences, and these untoward moldings that they go through along the way.

In response to an interview question asking faculty to describe a "low point" in their careers, many cited an experience of dishonesty. Faculty often described incidents of fraudulent or unethical behavior as examples of conflicts between their own values and the demands of a supervisor or the institutional leadership.

Dr. Haitham: I think the low points have to do with human relationships. Although research is what's exciting, I must say research failures haven't been low points in my life. I don't think they have bothered me. Failing research has never been a problem; I just think it comes with the territory. When I was younger and less secure, when experiments failed you did worry about it because how were you going to get the next grant funded? Those could be viewed as low points, in a shallow way. But the really low points were when I found the dishonesty . . . the lack of integrity in the system, and that in order to be successful you have to embrace that. I think it did depress me deeply, and I didn't know how I would ever survive in a system like this. . . . I think the way I did was to close off and just do what I wanted to do on a day to day basis. I lived without planning for the system, and I always had a job outside, so that any moment when things got unbearable I could just walk out. I think that's pretty low, [to be forced] to keep another job in your back pocket.

When I came, I wasn't young, but I was naïve. The level of dishonesty shocked me in terms of the need for control. People seemed to feel a tremendous need for control. I started learning that in a successful environment people succeed not only by doing well, they actually more often than not succeed by putting competitors down or out of business, by totally political means. This sounds absolutely incredible to most people. But perfectly bright people spent more of their time in politics and in strategizing success than actually doing anything. This may be much more peculiar to an institution like this, which is known for its success. Perhaps people feel more pressure to present themselves as more successful than they are, and perhaps that's what leads to moral corruption. At this stage in my life that still makes me feel pretty low. In fact, one of my goals is to not speak out, to be able to live with it, because you live with so much worse evil in life that you should be able to put up with it. I see resumes that are not quite true, and when I point it out to people, they say well it's not a lie, it may not be quite true. Because of that people obtained fairly high positions. The question is, do you want to spend the rest of your life aware of this?

Interviewer: You use this term "moral corruption" . . .

Dr. Haitham: Yeah. It is strong, but I think making up CVs is corrupt even if it's a minor change. I think taking a job and doing other things with your time, [without] accountability, is corruption. I think people get away with that a lot, but it's only the people who created this support system that do. And the group you will go to—to complain—are all part of the same system. It's like those mystery books where the victim goes and complains, and it turns out that the whole police department was part of the crime. That doesn't take away from the fact that this is a great institution, and I'm by and large extremely excited. And even these personalities have a tremendously valuable side; that's why it's much more depressing—there's no need for this kind of thing, but it does happen.

As Dr. Haitham's comment indicates, a major issue was that administrators and other people in authority were perceived to tolerate or even at times participate in unethical behavior.

One woman said that administrators tried to silence her when she brought to their attention a case of fraud, perhaps out of fear that making it public would tarnish the institution's reputation:

Another woman and I found that a doc was engaging in fraudulent research and in unethical behavior in his lab. The administration had asked our committee to review it. We completely concurred with the administration, and we wrote a joint report. I got hauled in to the vice president of medical affairs, who said that if he could, he'd fire me. He said that everything we said was true but we were "causing trouble."

Another complaint was that the institution refused to crack down on pharmaceutical company representatives promoting certain medications to students, residents, and attending physicians by buying their favor with expensive meals and "gifts" (a common practice in medical centers) or by paying for travel. Dr. Tonder commented:

We objected to the constant trail of drug reps coming in and feeding luncheons to the residents—time-honored tradition in the department.

Physicians are deluged with advertisements for medications and are given free samples of new expensive medications that can be administered to patients, usually at the initiation of a new treatment. This makes it much more likely that the physician will continue to prescribe the same medicine, even though it may have no advantage over older, well-tried, and cheaper medicines. The pharmaceutical companies actually track the prescribing habits of individual physicians to assess the effectiveness of their huge investments in marketing to the medical profession. Several studies have demonstrated that these marketing tactics are very effective in influencing physicians' choice of medications. Motivated by profit, industry proffers powerful inducements to influential faculty members to act as proponents of their products, such as new medications or medical devices, and often these inducements are not made public to institutions or patients. In 2009 a group of Harvard Medical School students demanded that pharmaceutical company support for educational programs be discontinued. The school convened a committee to discuss the issue, even though there already exists a substantial research literature documenting the unethical influence of pharmaceutical companies on students and physicians. Indeed, other medical schools had already adopted policies to address this evidence years earlier.

Many faculty were so disheartened by the whole spectrum of unethical practices they observed that they began to wonder whether they were in the right place. Dr. Peterson, a pediatrician, expressed a doubt many felt:

> Dr. Peterson: Maybe I am making different choices based on different things than the desire to advance in academic medicine, and why is that? Then you're asking, "Why am I here, why am I doing this, why am I doing it this way, if it is in opposition to things that I value?"

Dr. Westenfelder refused to compromise her integrity and left her institution:

> Dr. Westenfelder: I can work for somebody I don't like, but I refuse to work a long time for somebody I don't respect, and in fact, I think it was two months after this person [her supervisor] was appointed that I wrote my resignation letter and put it in my computer. I knew I would be using it at some time or other, but there were things that I wanted to accomplish, so it actually took two years before I eventually resigned. But I knew very early on that I wasn't going to work for this person long term. For me it was about what I needed to do to discharge my duty to the people I was leading.

Moral Distress and Women

Particularly striking in our interviews was how many women described discomfort with the disjuncture between their own values and those of their institution. They vehemently objected to some of the values they saw underlying their institution's actions. We also heard similar discomfort from men, but the disparity in values seemed particularly important to women who voiced their displeasure over this much more frequently. For example, twenty-two of twenty-six female leaders interviewed brought this up, whereas only seven of fourteen male leaders made similar comments.

Our results align with research findings by the social psychologist Shalom Schwartz, who in a series of cross-cultural studies found that women tend to value more than men qualities associated with benevolence and a sense of universalism (understanding, appreciation, tolerance, and protection for the welfare of all) (Schwartz and Rubel 2005). Our findings are also similar to those of Scott Wright and Brent Beasley at Johns Hopkins, who studied factors motivating internal medicine physician faculty (Wright and Beasley 2004). They found that female faculty were more motivated by helping others than were their male counterparts. Because women faculty place such a high value on others' welfare and the importance of helping, they are more likely to feel that the institution's social mission is imperative. This might explain why the women we interviewed felt greater discomfort or moral distress when they perceived that their institution was disregarding its social mission (Pololi et al. 2009).

These gender distinctions may shed some light on the question of why women have not achieved significant leadership positions in medical schools. As the next chapter will explain, the structure and culture of medical schools were developed by men at a time when there were no women in those institutions and are based on practices historically associated with men's life experiences. For these reasons, women are likely to be at a disadvantage in present medical school structure and culture.

Furthermore, when someone who feels she must always act according to her core values finds herself in a department with prevailing values that do not match her own, she is unable to fully meet that department's needs as its leaders see them, which means it will be difficult for her to advance professionally. An example is Dr. Tonder in Chapter 4, who was put in charge of faculty recruitment but refused to dissemble about what the department provided new faculty with. This contributed to Dr. Tonder's own moral distress, and as we saw, she eventually left academic medicine.

Many women described a leadership change in their institution that was accompanied by a shift in values as a major reason contributing to their dissatisfaction and in some cases their departure from academic medicine. Others left because they felt the work they were doing was not valued by the institution.

> Dr. Venetia: Now this is a. . . . key piece for me, this is the piece that changed. Initially I felt very much like a key part of the institution, and felt I was doing things that were important to me, and also important to the institution. And this changed over time. I no longer felt what was important to me was also important to the medical school. It got to the point where I felt I had to defend and justify what I was doing, that what I was doing was no longer important to the school.

Two other women leaders referred to a similar change in their institutions:

> Dr. Lilly: It was a matter of values changing in the school. Clearly it's linked to finances—we were in tight financial times and everything was being stripped down to the essentials. Some of the things I had been working on were considered to no longer be essential. They were more peripheral. Teamwork became less valued, interdisciplinary teamwork in particular was less valued, and people who were considered adjunct, as educators are, were seen as not full partners anymore. And I think that was a key piece.

> Dr. Sanders: I think that in my ten years there I was able to define a niche where my personal values could be expressed and aligned with a portion of the institution. So it was possible to stay there and to be productive and to enjoy it. I don't think that my personal values aligned with the overall institutional values, and I think ultimately that's why I left.

Authenticity and Betrayal of Trust

This chapter has described what faculty perceived as several forms of betrayal—of the public trust in the medical school's social mission to patients and the community; of its obligation to educate future physicians not only in knowledge, but also to be principled, ethical, and idealistic; and of faculty members' trust in their colleagues and leaders. These betrayals have consequences not only for medical faculty's personal and professional lives but for their overall effectiveness and for what faculty can contribute to their institutions.

Key to the question of values-conflict is the concept of authenticity. This has been described as a characteristic of people who act in accordance with their values, preferences, and needs as opposed to acting merely to please others, attain rewards, or avoid punishments (Goldmann and Kernis 2002). In practice, this means that people who can freely express their own feelings, thoughts, and beliefs at their workplace can bring more of their selves to their roles and are more deeply engaged in what they are doing (Kahn 1990, 1992). It is then that they are best able to create connections with one another that can bridge differences such as gender, race, and ethnicity and form trusting relationships (Alderfer 1987). And it is within these relationships that they can work through difficulties, resulting in growth and learning (Smith and Berg 1987).

A related insight comes from Mihaly Csikszentmihalyi's studies on "flow," a term he uses to refer to the state of operating at the peak of one's abilities, experiencing both total concentration and deep enjoyment. His work shows that people who find their lives meaningful usually have a goal that is challenging enough to take up all their energies, a goal that can give joyful and important significance to their lives (Csikszentmihalyi 2000). Ideally, we would like medical faculty to be functioning in a "flow" state. It is when this purposeful optimal activity is applied to what they value most deeply that faculty can be most successful and satisfied. Certainly our interviews make it clear that faculty enjoy striving to meet crucial challenges and being resolute in pursuing an important goal. What is more, faculty are much more likely to instill a passion for humanistic care in their students or conduct stellar research when working on something they feel passionate about.

In essence, then, we want faculty to be authentic at work—not only believing that their personal values align with those of the workplace but knowing also that they can be themselves there. Three simple examples exemplify the type of benefit that would ensue. The first involves a faculty member, Dr. Southie, who grew up in a family of social activists.

Dr. Southie felt passionately and doggedly that service to the community and the underserved was a responsibility and that it should be incorporated into training programs of health professions at a time when this was quite unusual. Dr. Southie took a number of professional risks to stay true to this personal commitment. Her efforts resulted in some outstanding underserved community-based training programs that were eventually fully recognized and supported, as well as in the providing of transformative learning experiences for the students involved.

Dr. Amica had a child with a learning disability. To ensure that her child could perform well in school, Dr. Amica learned a great deal about how to recognize and manage this particular disability. At the medical school, she was on a committee to assess students experiencing academic difficulties. The committee found itself dealing with problems Dr. Amica was able to identify as learning disabilities. In this way, she brought the expertise developed to help her own child—an issue emotionally dear to her—into her workplace. Soon, Dr. Amica became known and respected as someone with valuable knowledge in this area. Being able to bring that important part of herself to work and having it valued made her feel that she had more of a place in the school and gave her work more meaning. It also greatly contributed to the effectiveness of the educational program and to the outcomes for students, who now received the help they needed.

Under different circumstances, Dr. Amica might have been afraid to let her colleagues know she had this particular problem in her life, since in many medical schools it is not common to open up about one's home life or express concern about one's children; there would be an assumption that personal or family problems were distractions preventing one from being fully dedicated to the job. The same might be true for expressions of emotion about other events in one's life outside the workplace such as a divorce or one's own illness. Being respected in such a competitive workplace usually requires walling off everything else that is important in one's personal life.

A third example is a pediatric surgeon with a passion for amateur photography. Many of Dr. Sprague's patients came from underprivileged and immigrant families. When a child needed surgery, the parents were often quite fearful. They did not understand the procedure and were afraid that the child would not recover fully. The surgeon began taking photos of the young patients before surgery and giving them to the parents. Dr. Sprague found that the photos were tremendously important to the parents, most of whom had no photos of their children. She also found that she could reduce the anxiety of apprehensive parents by showing them photographs of other children taken after successful surgeries. Taking these photos became a regular practice. Some time later, Dr. Sprague created exhibitions of these photographs as well as pictures she took of other aspects of medicine. Her photography thus became part of her professional identity, and she began giving talks about it around the country.

Making photography part of Dr. Sprague's work life enhanced her profile within her institution and made her feel more successful. Because she was at a school where she had no need to hide that personal interest, she was able to become known for something outside of medical skills or accomplishments. If—as happens elsewhere—she had been reluctant to let her colleagues know about her private interests, the great benefit her photography brought to her, her patients, and her institution would have been lost.

Medical faculty functioning at the peak of their abilities may be the most precious resource in the nation's medical schools. Given the high levels of dissatisfaction, burnout, and turnover in medical faculty nationwide, it is important to explore the factors preventing them from being authentic at work. The more of their real selves they can bring to their workplace, the more meaning they may experience, particularly in those tasks that demand more of them at a personal level. By the same token, institutions must respond to their faculty's stated personal values. For example, if someone believes that education is an important institutional mission and responsibility, she needs to have time to do that well, and her successful efforts must be earnestly recognized and rewarded. Similarly, if a faculty member wants to address a need in the local community or collaborate in a research project in the community, this too needs to be recognized and included in the reward system, as should any resulting scholarship.

If the institution makes it difficult for faculty to act according to their core values, the medical faculty cannot be authentic and make their optimal contribution. The institution loses the full abilities of the people on its payroll, and the faculty themselves are unhappy and might leave. What is clear not only from the existing research on authenticity but also from our own interviews is that, when the heart does not feel honored, we do not do our best work—"heart" here meaning the core place within ourselves where all our faculties converge—will, intellect, intuition, and feelings (Palmer 2003).

REFERENCES

Alderfer CP. An intergroup perspective on group dynamics. In: Lorsch JW, ed. Handbook of organizational behavior. Englewood Cliffs, NJ: Prentice-Hall; 1987:190–222.

Bogue EG. An agenda of common caring: the call for community in higher education. In: McDonald W, ed. Creating campus community: in search of Ernest Boyer's legacy. San Francisco: Jossey-Bass; 2002:1–19.

Cohen JJ, Siegel EK. Academic medical centers and medical research: the challenges ahead. JAMA. 2005;294:1367–72.

Csikszentmihalyi M. Beyond boredom and anxiety: experiencing flow in work and play. San Francisco: Jossey-Bass; 2000:216.

Goldman BM, Kernis MH. The role of authenticity in healthy psychological functioning and subjective well-being. Ann Am Psychother Assoc. 2002;5(6): 18–20.

Kahn WA. Psychological conditions of personal engagement and disengagement at work. Acad Management J. 1990;33:692–724.

Kahn WA. To be fully there: psychological presence at work. Hum Relat. 1992 45:321–49.

Martinson BC, Anderson MS, de Vries R. Scientists behaving badly. Nature. 2005;435:737–8.

Palmer PJ. Honor and the human heart. Natl Staff Dev Council. 2003;24:49–53.

Pololi L, Dennis K, Mitchell JA. A needs assessment of medical school faculty: Caring for the caretakers. J Contin Educ Health Prof. 2003;23:21–9.

Pololi L, Kern DE, Carr P, Conrad P, Knight S. The culture of academic medicine: faculty perceptions of the lack of alignment between individual and institutional values. J Gen Intern Med. 2009;24(12):1289–95.

Schwartz SH, Rubel T. Sex differences in value priorities: cross-cultural and multi-method studies. J Pers Soc Psychol. 2005;89(6):1010–28.

Smith KK, Berg DN. Paradoxes of group life: understanding conflict, paralysis, and movement in group dynamic. San Francisco: Jossey-Bass; 1987.

Wright SM, Beasley BW. Motivating factors for academic physicians within departments of medicine. Mayo Clin Proc. 2004;79:1145–50.

Chapter 6 Dual Vision: Women Faculty and Medical Culture

> There seems to have been a race between our becoming, for example, profes-
> sors [or doctors], and our sufficiently changing the world for it to be morally
> acceptable for us to occupy such positions. This was not, of course, a race we
> could win; we were, that is, doomed to succeed (those of us who did succeed,
> and, of course, not all did) more quickly than we could change the world. We
> told ourselves, in part, that we were succeeding precisely in order to have the
> power to change the world, but the result is that we have become, structurally,
> "them." The moral questions we now face turn not on purity (hopelessly un-
> available to us) but on acceptable, politically accountable, compromise: can
> we live the positions we occupy differently enough? —Naomi Scheman (1993)

Women faculty's predominant response to our interview questions was to describe the richness of their professional lives and to emphasize how much they loved their work. It was this very deep satisfaction and sense of privilege at being able to do this work that kept them in their jobs. By and large, not unlike male faculty, they appreciated the many positive aspects of being medical school faculty and tolerated the less congenial aspects of medical school culture. Still, they also pointed to a number of difficulties that they experienced specifically *as women*. Although men too were affected by the competitiveness, disconnection, and erosion of trust described in Chapters 4 and 5, the women experienced medical school culture differently. This was partly because they brought a different set of life experiences to their workplace and partly because they felt they were treated differently.

Whereas men were more likely to express an unqualified feeling of belonging to their institutions, women felt marginalized and invisible. They felt excluded from the "male culture" of the medical school; they sometimes faced active discrimination as well as nonconscious bias; and they sometimes felt self-doubt. Women often feel like outsiders in medical school culture, and in this respect they resemble other outsiders, especially members of groups that are underrepresented in medicine, such as African Americans and Latinos.

Feeling Marginalized and Invisible

Women felt marginalized and invisible both because there were so few of them and because they felt like cultural outsiders in the organization of academic medicine. This feeling of invisibility, or being ignored, may be a cardinal marker of marginalization.

Few Women in Leadership

Interviewees said it was unusual to see other women in leadership positions and that the actual leaders, who were almost exclusively male, seemed to have little interest in women assuming positions of authority. Dr. Rouge, an accomplished faculty member in a psychiatry department, explained that the lack of women in leadership roles in her department resulted in a "male culture." She described her frustration over this invisibility. Because women were not visible as leaders, they were less noticed when current faculty members were being considered or new ones sought for promotions. They were also not asked to speak at meeting presentations.

> Dr. Rouge: Everybody who's in charge is a guy—the chief, the next-to-chief, and the head of all the subdepartments. Even the clinical head of my subdivision is a guy. And all these women with doctorates certainly are more qualified than he is. It isn't like he's brilliant either; he's tall but he's no rocket scientist. And it throws me that they would put him in charge. I can't imagine what they see as his qualifications. He looks like them, and I do think when men are in charge they often have a vision of who else is going to move into those spots, and they're often people who look like them, and it's not necessarily even conscious prejudice. If I imagine certain roles, a woman pops into mind for me, so it's not surprising.
>
> And when they sit at the front and they're presenting, they make eye contact with each other—they don't make eye contact with you; if you

raise your hand, they don't call on you. If they have a committee to plan what is going to happen, they don't ask you to be on it. So I guess that's a male culture. Not to mention that all the secretaries are always women. The whole support net structure is always women.

Describing one of the regular case presentations held in her department, Dr. Rouge noted:

I just wanted to scream—they trotted the same men out and said the same things they say every week. No women on the panel. It wasn't a woman presenting the case. The case wasn't about a woman. I put my hand up to comment on the case, and I couldn't get called on. Afterward, I went up to them and said, "What do I have to do to get called on?" They were not expecting that.

Many interviewees commented on the absence of women leaders. Dr. Jones, a midcareer physician, made it clear that she missed having female role models:

I have never been in a position where I saw any women in power. . . . I did not see any women who were successful in the sense that they were both professors and had families. . . . I've never had a [female] colleague onsite who had similar enough interests where we could really talk about science.

Dr. Schmidt, a primary care physician: All the second tier leaders are women; not a single one of the first tier leaders are. [chuckles] Women are definitely underrepresented in leadership here.

Women in male-dominated specialties especially felt the lack of significant numbers of women in their departments. Dr. Cooper, an obstetrician, reflected on the difficulty of her early years in this male-dominated field, which has since become much more diverse, and even majority female.

Dr. Cooper: When I first came here, the face of the department was very different. I was one of the only females in the department. There had never been a female faculty member that had become pregnant during the course of being here. Everyone was full time, everyone had an at-home wife that was taking care of them, so I felt like an outsider. I didn't feel a part of it, and I didn't feel particularly supported. As time has gone on, now predominantly it's women in the field. And we have a department of twenty, and half of the faculty are women, and we also have much more diversity than we had before. We have African-American people, we have gays and lesbians, and we have just more women in general, so that the face of the department, to me at least, seems more welcoming and more like there's room to be yourself rather than having to fit into a mold.

Dr. Frederick, a senior scientist, echoed Dr. Cooper's sentiment, but her feeling of marginalization was current:

> I'm female in a very male specialty and male environment. Fewer than 10 percent of the ——ists in this country are female. So, many times I am an outsider.

When asked whether she hoped to one day feel "part of the cliques" that she observed among the physicians in her department, Dr. Frederick quipped: "No. I'm not a guy. I don't play golf."

Dr. Brown experienced a double outsider status as an African-American woman:

> What I struggled with for a long time here was my being an African-American woman in a white, male-dominated institution, and the feeling that I was invisible. . . . I wasn't counted; my opinion didn't matter; what I was feeling didn't matter. I felt like that for at least the first ten years. There were people who I passed every single day, who were chairmen of departments, and I mean, good God, after five years you've got to see a person . . . Yet they never acknowledged my presence. And I often thought it was a reflection of my race, to be honest with you. Okay, being a woman has to do with it too, but I think these just are racist people. They maybe don't know how to talk to me because I'm an African-American person.

She summarized the painful and disorienting effects of this invisibility:

> Dr. Brown: It's too hard to feel invisible for a long time. How much can you take? Maybe the only reason I stayed is because I didn't think I had

a lot of options . . . It's very difficult to be marginalized and made to feel that you're not important . . . not a whole lot of people understand what that really feels like.

A midcareer woman in an administrative role described the lack of interest on the part of department chairs when a nationally recognized speaker came to her medical school to make a presentation about the advancement of women in medicine. The reactions of the chairs marginalized the entire issue of women in medicine in a number of ways.

> Dr. Geordino: We decided to have an expert on women's issues do presentations the whole day, for the medical students, for faculty and staff, etc. She has a talk she gives for administrators and department chairs, a management toolbox. She is extremely knowledgeable. The dean had a whole series of leadership trainings for the department chairs, but the dean never did announce this. Finally, as he was getting ready to dismiss the chairs' group prior to her visit, I said I'd like to announce that the next chairs' group will be her presentation. The men department chairs, which are the majority, kind of frowned at each other and some of them rolled their eyes, like, "What's this, and what are we being expected to come to?" When she arrived, folks were slow to arrive. Only about half the department chairs showed up, and they acted like my little brother used to act when my mother would drag him to my violin recital. [laughs] Like they were forced to be there, but they didn't want to be there. She presented excellent information. But anything viewed as something for women, they don't want to have anything to do with it. We have a long way to go.

Cultural Outsiders

Women do not feel part of the bonhomie and mutually supportive male leadership groups in medical schools. They find themselves excluded in ways ranging from minor cultural habits to significant policies.

Dr. Frederick reported a typical instance of seemingly unconscious exclusion when a "fellow" (a physician doing advanced clinical training after residency) was not assigned a sufficient number of clinical patients (or cases) to manage.

> Dr. Frederick: We just had an issue in the lab this past year where we had a female fellow who just wasn't being given cases. . . . They just picked the guy they knew best or who was convenient and at hand instead of distributing cases equally among all the fellows. . . . I don't think it was deliberate. . . . It's just like, oh my bud is right here. You know the guy who was a fellow with us and didn't come from the outside, [whom] they knew better, was just right here.

Dr. Haitham, a senior scientist in a leadership position, described how, despite her position and authority, she still felt like an outsider, since her interests and values were so different from those of the relatively elite leadership group. The faculty lacked diversity, and no one shared her interest in developing programs for poor people. As a result, she felt she did not fit in, was not interested in their talk, and never mixed socially.

> Dr. Haitham: I haven't made an effort to become more a part of the system. I [used to] think of it as part of my job, to be in that leadership group, but no more. And I think part of it really does have to do with the fact that I'm a woman, a different ethnicity. So for example within the leadership, there are within the center about 150 people; I don't think I feel that much part of the system. Again, I don't socialize with anyone because that's where the value systems are different.

Dr. Sanders, a woman of color, described how her isolation made it difficult to understand the reality of what was happening around her:

> Early on there were just no women and certainly no faculty of color . . . you are by yourself, and you don't have the test group of reality-oriented—the kind of people you can say listen, this happened, what do you think is going on—where there's a commonality of experiences. I think it's true both from the dynamics of gender and race. There are some things that happen that clearly are driven by race, other things that happen that are driven by gender, and then some where you never know. But when you're by yourself, you don't have someone else to reflect from.

Women's sense of being ignored exists not necessarily because male leaders consciously set out to exclude women but because historically, the organizational structure and practices of academic medicine were largely created and developed by men for men. As a result, many of the norms of academic medical culture were developed around men's work habits and propensities. Professors Robin Ely and Debra Meyerson from Harvard and Stanford, scholars in management sciences, have written lucidly about the ways that policies and interactions that appear gender-neutral because they are the norms of organizational life do in fact disadvantage women. In this section, I draw heavily on their insightful work.

As Ely and Meyerson note, "The social practices in these organizations tend to reflect and support men's life experiences" (Ely and Meyerson 2000). These supposedly gender-neutral practices and policies actually reward and support particular masculine characteristics and behaviors. For example, assertiveness, independence, individualism, and competitiveness are associated with male socialization in Western cultures, so that male development is generally tied to expectations of individuality, leadership, and hierarchy.

Thus, to take one important institutional practice, the criteria for granting tenure, which depends on requesting the advancement, self-promotion, and autonomous performance, all favor male behavior patterns. Ely and Meyerson also point out the persistence of the historical theme that man's role is to provide for the family by working in the public sphere and woman's role is to work in the private realm as mother. This legacy translates into an assumption that the ideal worker is willing and able to prioritize work over all other activities, and that real "commitment" means unrestricted availability—putting family obligations second to work obligations. Although this expectation applies to everyone and as such appears gender-neutral, it penalizes those who are unable to be available at all times—which is to say women, since in our culture women frequently bear a disproportionate responsibility for dependent care and will suffer the most when they are unable to meet this expectation. Women who are single parents are particularly disadvantaged. As Ely and Meyerson note, "A close look at these practices reveals implicit gender bias that maintains women's relative disadvantage" (Ely and Meyerson 2000).

Another sociologist, Joan Acker, dissected dimensions of social relations into four categories: formal policies and procedures; informal work practices, norms, and patterns of work; narratives, language, and symbolic expressions; and informal patterns of everyday social interaction (Acker 1990). Our interviews offer examples of how women are excluded in all these categories.

Some interviewees (usually in their thirties or forties), attempting to combine a rich professional life with caring for young children, commented on the difficulties of doing this. Two midcareer women described how ambitious and competent women with young children felt ambivalent about taking on leadership positions because of time constraints.

> Dr. Silverman: So women who are five to ten years younger than me are now largely in the young child stage of their family life, and they are all paralyzed by ambivalence. They're ambitious and they're competent and they're wonderful [small laugh], but when it comes to being offered any kind of opportunity to take leadership—those [opportunities] they can't afford.

Dr. Flower, a generalist faculty member, explained her own ambivalence:

> So I guess I dabbled with it [leadership]. I struggle with, maybe I really should do more of it, but I'm not sure I'm that good at it. I don't know. . . . If it goes well it's fun. I've got some ideas that I think would be very useful in improving the health care of the people of [her state] and improving the efficiency of the university, but I've also had three kids that really needed my attention.

Dr. Knight, a gynecologist, received pointed comments from her colleagues because her behavior confounded their stereotypical assumption that her "gender appropriate" role as a mother was more important than her aspirations as a researcher. Dr. Knight had accepted a part-time salary in exchange for having one day free to pursue her own research. However, she quickly discovered that her colleagues "did not have the same vision of academics" as she did and thought of her one (nonclinical) research day as her "free day." Not only was her role as a researcher not valued in this department, but some of her colleagues were judgmental about her choice and quite sexist in their responses to her work. She recalled bumping into one colleague, whom she considered a friend at the time, after she got off a clinical call shift. He asked: "So what are you going to do today? Are you going to do your research stuff or are you going to go home and love your kid?"

> Dr. Knight: I had a one-year old at home at the time. I didn't say anything, but you can imagine the expletives that were going on in my mind, be-

cause in my mind, the most important work—my critical day—was the time that I was not seeing patients.

When Carol Greider was interviewed on winning the 2009 Nobel Prize in Physiology or Medicine for work on telomeres, she was asked "Do this year's Nobels mean that women have finally been accepted in science?" Dr. Greider replied: "I certainly hope that it's a sign that things are going to be different in the future. I'm a scientist, right? I'm not going to see one event and say it's a trend. One of the things I did with the press conference that Johns Hopkins gave was to have my two kids there. In the newspaper, there's a picture of me and my kids right there. How many men have won the Nobel in the last few years, and they have kids the same age as mine, and their kids aren't in the picture?" (Dreifus 2009). In the interview, there was never a hint of work-family conflict, but rather of Dr. Greider's deep excitement and fulfillment through her career in science and her awareness that projecting her identity both as scientist and parent is unusual in the culture of academic medicine.

A related disadvantage for women is that one prerequisite for promotion is travel and presenting at meetings. Some interviewees mentioned that this expectation limited their ability to advance. Dr. Sanders, who was a successful senior physician, said:

> I think one of the reasons women don't get promoted as much in academia is because we are not willing to travel as much, and that's something I worry a whole lot about. In order to get promoted you . . . have to attend meetings, be willing to give talks. And women tend not to be able to do that because of family obligations. I've been willing to do that, but there is always a price. My child misses me. My husband wants to know how much I have to travel. I think that's going to be a real problem, as we go forward trying to have women be part of the infrastructure. The way it's set up is that you travel, you're around, you're mobile. Women actually were better prepared to help men do that versus men helping women do that. The women I know who are in academia—the travel is the hardest part. It's being able to do the traveling, [and] be available for everybody and to juggle all that at once.

This disadvantage too grows out of the historical "male culture" in which men could travel because there was always a woman taking care of home and children.

Another cultural difference arises because organizations in Western cultures value individualism over communality and collaboration. The system rests on belief in the value of individual merit and achievement, and its reward systems reflect this belief. Whereas individualism and competitiveness are associated with manliness, collaboration and communality are associated with womanliness. Accordingly, collaboration is not rewarded in the current promotion and tenure systems of academic medicine. In fact, collaboration is considered an indication that one may be unable to perform independently.

Two senior women described the cultural gap between themselves and the men they worked with in terms of men's socialization playing team sports.

> Dr. Skinner: Many women never learned—it's not so much the team stuff, it's the point that you have to be willing to get on the field, get knocked down by some 250[-pound] hulk who's going to do something dirty, you know, creepy, to you and then you have to be able to go out and be his chum or at least make the appearance of being his chum again. And girls don't get that training. . . . That hurts women, all the kind of old boy networks that we just don't have. So when committees or advisory boards are thought of, the boys think of the boys, and they very rarely recommend a woman.

> Dr. Tonder: I'd never played team sports or I had never dealt with male group behavior. I was used to saying what I thought. I was used to people arguing on the basis of the issues, not having all kinds of political sub-agendas. I was very naïve, and I didn't have a mentor. My own chairman was terribly good at that kind of game-playing, so I mean I ended up being pretty good at it, but I hated it. And because I was often the only woman or one of only a couple [of] women, the men were willing to take liberties in terms of ad hominem attacks that they would never take with each other.

Stereotypes and Symbols

As Acker points out, stories, symbols, and language in frequent use all help codify "the way things are." For example, women feel uncomfortable and "out of the game" when men get together, put their feet up on the table, and pepper their talk with allusions to sports. Dr. Geordino, an administrator, gave an example of how the habits of male culture have a marginalizing, alienating effect on women.

> The previous dean had a group he called the Dean's Council, which had not only the department heads which were all male, but also the assistant dean and directors of different programs. There were about three or four women who attended the meeting. When the new dean came in, I think the department chairs asked to have it be made a chairs' group only, and for a time it was only men; there were no women there. Some of the women came to me and complained that even though we thought the dean was supportive of women, the medical school was becoming less and less of a friendly place for women to work, and information was not trickling down as it should. So I talked to the dean about that and he said, "Well, you start coming."
>
> We now have two women chairs, which has been helpful. If they'd been to some meeting about battling for funding, they'd come back and report on that and talk about "Spraying testosterone around the table," it's just a big joke.
>
> This [was] an issue of great hilarity. We were getting ready to hire a woman chair, and I made a comment about it. And [the dean] said, "Oh . . . we're just joking, and it's making fun of us. It's not meant to be exclusive." He just couldn't see that it was exclusionary. But they stopped making offensive jokes because we had women as department chairs. But it's just a completely different culture and we're seen, as women, as the ones that "don't fit", in my experience.

Many research studies have described stereotypic thinking or "gender schemas," consisting of numerous nonconscious hypotheses about differences between women and men. As Virginia Valian noted, gender schemas play a central role in shaping men's and women's professional lives. They "affect our expectations of men and women, our evaluations of their work, and their performance as professionals" (Valian 1998). Alice Eagly argues that women are socialized to emphasize similarities and connections, or, as it is sometimes called, communality (Eagly 1987; Eagly and Carli 2007). When women behave in communal ways, they are rewarded in society generally with reinforcement of gender stereotypic behavior.

The widely held perception of these differences becomes a widespread assumption of fixed, innate differences between men and women—for example, that men are more aggressive and women are more emotional and relational. This gender schema often influences the way men and women are evaluated. Thus if a woman does not meet performance expectations based on a masculine framework of competence, her failure is construed as confirming the stereotype, and she receives less benefit of the doubt than her male counterparts. For example, Dr. Geordino perceived different sets of standards for men and women that were informed by performance expectations shaped by gender schemas.

> Dr. Geordino: It's not unique to our institution: if a man is in a position and somebody considers that he screwed up in some way, they'll try to work it out, to help him. If a woman does the same thing, there's usually a head shaking, tsk-tsking. . . . "We should have known that she couldn't handle this."

By the same token, when a woman's behavior conforms to the female stereotype—for example if she puts time into nurturing juniors—she receives little reward, since feminine competencies are less valued than masculine competencies. Helping others develop their potential is considered "nice but not necessary." Consequently, the emphasis on promoting one's own achievements—which requires getting fast results to demonstrate to others—winds up discouraging people from nurturing others and from building systems that are needed to sustain and advance the organization in the long term. As one woman quoted in Chapter 4 noted, women may get praise for helping others become better clinicians, but the institution does not value this work, so they must do it on their own time.

Not only are women devalued for acting in "feminine" ways, they also find themselves in the very difficult situation of paying a price for behavior that is stereotypically "male," such as being tough and assertive (Costrich et al. 1975; Rudman 1998; Heilman 2001; Eagly and Carli 2007). Advancing in organizations depends not only on assessment of competence but also on social acceptance. The combination of receiving a lower evaluation for similar performance and behaving in ways that are stereotypically male (violating the norms of how women "should" behave) constitutes a potent set of barriers that women must confront as they advance in an organization.

A series of studies by Madeline Heilman, a professor of psychology at New York University, demonstrated that success in traditionally male-dominated jobs often has negative consequences for women, including social rejection and disapproval (Heilman 2004). For example, successful female employees were significantly less liked than equally successful male employees in a typically male job such as a management position, whereas they were judged more likable in a typically female job. Additionally, women in traditionally male positions are often on the receiving end of derogatory personal characterizations such as "battle axe," "ice queen," and "bitch." Heilman concluded that her results help explain why "despite their success, high powered women often tend to not advance to the very top levels of organizations" (Heilman 2004). Her studies help explain why women are perceived as "not a good fit" in the club of upper management and leadership, where perceived negative personal qualities would result in rejection.

Marianne La France studied conversational behavior and interruptions across gender. Her research demonstrated that conversational interruptions that occurred among mixed-sex pairs (but not in same-sex pairs) are often interpreted as disrespectful behavior in women (but less so in men) and an assault on established power relations. When a woman interrupts a man, she has broken more than a conversational rule; she has impugned an accepted social prescript concerning appropriate behavior by those possessing less power. Interruptions in this context connote impertinence rather than contentiousness (LaFrance 1992).

Laurie Rudman of Rutgers University showed that, in settings where self-promotion was important for getting hired or promoted, women who behaved confidently and assertively were not as well received as men who behaved similarly. Generally women who promoted themselves were assessed as more competent, but at the same time were considered less likable and less hireable (Rudman 1998). Chapter 7 will discuss further how women in leadership positions suffer because of stereotypic thinking.

Ely and Meyerson comment that "men may acknowledge a woman's ability to act like men with such compliments as 'she kicks ass with the best of them' or 'she's hard as nails,' but these compliments cut two ways. "While they provide some positive recognition for a woman's ability to mobilize competitive masculinity, they also serve as strong remind-

ers . . . that [women] have violated social norms associated with feminin-
ity and thereby raise questions about their status as women" (Ely and
Meyerson 2000).

Even though much of this research on nonconscious bias is not new
and is well known to social scientists, it is still relevant and in fact has
only just been applied to academic medicine. Professor Molly Carnes at
the University of Wisconsin has been a real pioneer in this effort (Carnes
et al. 2005). This wealth of empirical research shows that women's experiences of bias in academic medicine, as demonstrated in our interviews,
reflect more general phenomena. The effect of all these forms of marginalization is to suppress a range of approaches that women (and other
marginalized groups) could bring to academic medical centers and patient outcomes. The result of this marginalization of women could in the
long term be a disadvantage to the institution.

Active Discrimination

Beyond the more or less unconscious biases described above, some women
(and minority faculty members as well) experienced active discrimination, which reinforced their outsider status in their departments or institutions. A significant source of this discrimination is the often expressed
bias that women have less ability in science than men. This notion persists not only among the public at large but at the highest levels of the
science community. There has been hot debate in the popular press, at
universities, and in schools about whether girls and women are as good
as boys and men in mathematics and science. The dedication to science
so apparent in comments by our interviewees stands in sharp contrast to
this prejudice. Research clearly proves that women's scientific and mathematical abilities are equal to men's. Mathematics is at the heart of all
science and technology, and (to take one example) Leahey and Guo reported in 2001 that mathematics test scores were almost identical among
20,000 U.S. boys and girls between the ages of 4 and 18 (Leahey and Guo
2001). Professors Janet Hyde and Janet Mertz at the University of Wisconsin, Madison, also showed that in the United States, girls and boys
perform equally well on standardized mathematics tests at all levels. They
also concluded from their studies that changeable sociocultural factors,
not innate biological differences between the sexes, lead to gender in-

equality and are the primary reasons for fewer females than males being identified as excelling in mathematics at the highest levels in most countries (Hyde and Mertz 2009).

In 2005, Harvard University president Larry Summers pondered whether innate differences could account for women's failure to advance in the sciences. This view was further developed by Harvard professor Harvey Mansfield in *Manliness,* where he asserts that women do not like to compete; are less abstract thinkers; are risk averse; and are too emotional (Mansfield 2006). Harvard cognitive scientist Steven Pinker also argued that innate differences explain the reduced numbers of successful female scientists. But female Harvard scientists were not convinced. Elizabeth Spelke, a prominent psychologist, her colleagues, and many other researchers have shown that talented girls and boys demonstrate equal aptitude for mathematics by the most meaningful measures. There is no rigorous scientific evidence supporting the notion that women are more emotional or less competitive than men, and—despite widely read pop science claims—other studies show no gender differences in communication. Medical school assessments indicate that women entering careers in academic medicine are equally well prepared and accomplished as men.

Nevertheless this bias persists at the highest levels. It was evident in 2004, when the National Institutes of Health did not award a single one of nine prestigious research grants to a woman. A review of the process noted that sixty of the sixty-four evaluators of the submitted proposals were men and that the nominating process seemed to favor male applicants. The entire incident demonstrated a clear lack of awareness of bias against women in the sciences, such as in evaluation of proposals, and an absence of intent to address the lack of women in the sciences. Although NIH did change its procedures and increasingly awarded grants to women in subsequent years, many studies illustrate pervasive unconscious bias against women in research science careers. In 2008, Timothy Ley published a report examining gender differences in NIH grantee awards. He found that the percentage of successfully funded proposals was significantly lower for women than for men for those submitted by senior women for competing renewals of RO1s and women MDs submitting their first RO1 (Ley and Hamilton 2008).

Our interview data agree with these findings and other research that clearly shows gender discrimination. Several recent studies document overt forms of discrimination in medical schools. Research collaborators of mine, Professors Phyllis Carr and Arlene Ash of Boston University, and Brandeis colleague Rosalind Chait Barnett, conducted a 1995 survey of over 3,000 faculty in U.S. medical schools and found that female faculty were 2.5 times more likely than male faculty to perceive gender discrimination in the academic environment. Among women, rates of reported discrimination ranged from 47 percent for the youngest faculty to 70 percent for the oldest. About half of the female faculty but few male faculty had experienced some form of sexual harassment. Female faculty who reported being sexually harassed also perceived gender-specific bias in the academic environment more often than did other women (80 percent compared with 61 percent) and more often reported experiencing gender bias in professional advancement (72 percent compared with 47 percent) (Carr et al. 2000). Another study showed that 40 percent of a group of women medical faculty interviewed ranked gender discrimination first out of eleven possible choices for hindering their careers (Carr et al. 2003).

Rhea Steinpreis and colleagues at the University of Wisconsin in Milwaukee studied factors that influenced outside reviewers and search committee members when they were reviewing curricula vitae (CV) for recruitment purposes. The researchers used a single CV from a real female scientist but changed the name to an obviously male one on half the copies. Both men and women evaluators who reviewed these CVs were more likely to hire the male applicant than the female applicant. Similarly, both male and female evaluators reported that the male job applicant had more adequate teaching, research, and service experience compared with the female applicant—even though the records were identical (Steinpreis et al. 1999)! Steinpreis and other researchers suggest that such bias results in women being less likely to be hired (Steinpreis et al. 1999; Biernat and Fuegen 2001; Heilman et al. 2004; Uhlmann and Cohen 2005).

Among biomedical faculty, women receive less favorable letters of recommendation and peer review of their scientific articles (Trix and Penska 2003; Wenneras and Wold 1997). Frances Trix and Carolyn Penska, anthropologists from Wayne State University, examined more than 300 letters of recommendation for medical faculty at a large U.S. medical school in the mid-1990s. Letters written for female applicants differed systematically from those written for male applicants in terms of length, in the higher percentages of terms used that raised doubts, and in the lower frequency of mention of status terms, such as "research" or scientific terminology. The language used also reinforced gender schemas that portrayed women as teachers and students, and men as researchers and professionals (Trix and Penska 2003). Women are also sparsely represented on the editorial boards of biomedical science journals (Keiser et al. 2003; Jagsi et al. 2008).

Further supporting evidence of the pervasiveness of gender bias in science comes from Sweden. Christine Wenneras' and Agnes Wold's study is remarkable because Sweden is ranked by the United Nations as the leading country in the world with respect to equal opportunities for men and women. Gender equity is firmly embedded in the social structures of Sweden, which mandates that the legislature and corporate boards include specified proportions of women. Even so, an investigation of discrimination against women there was prompted by the fact that the success rate for female scientists applying for postdoctoral fellowships was half that of male applicants. In a study of the peer-review system of a major national funding agency for biomedical research, Wenneras found that women needed to be judged two and a half times as productive (as measured by their research publications) as men to be considered equally competent. The reviewers gave female applicants lower average scores than male applicants on all three evaluation parameters: scientific competence, quality of the proposed methodology, and relevance of the research proposal. It is also the first such study based on actual peer-review scores; the authors had to go to court to be able to see them. This study "strongly suggested that peer reviewers cannot judge scientific merit independent of gender."

Dr. Booker, a prominent scientist, described in detail her own inequitable treatment despite considerable achievements at a very prestigious university. She was not given appropriate status or lab space for her work. Her efforts were marginalized, and she needed the intervention of her husband, who was on the faculty, and a new chairman to achieve her potential (and eventually highly successful) outcomes.

I did not feel very much like I belonged to my department or was at the university. But part of that was because I started at a marginalized position. When I began to research as an independent PI [principal investigator], I was on a nontenure-track position, which is a not uncommon path for women. Most women don't progress beyond that, and I don't believe that is because of their abilities, but because it's not a position that is structured to allow you to progress beyond it. [I got] lots of support from my husband and [had] success with students, because I happened to be in a department where there were really no viable women (there was one woman faculty member, but she didn't have students). So I was the only alternative for students who were looking for something that they couldn't get from the male faculty—or I shouldn't say the male faculty—the other faculty members. I got a group of graduate students who felt that they weren't good enough to get PhD's, which is ridiculous I might add, and so it benefited me. I had the opportunity to be an independent PI. Because it was a relatively small department where there was an abundant student population, I was able to get graduate students, not very many, but you don't need very many. I built a little community with my students—I might add, they weren't all women, but most of them were—so I belonged with my group. But I never was able to create any kinds of ties within the department, partly a function of the fact that these departments are notorious for not being very welcoming.

Interviewer: Why did you feel that you didn't belong, that you weren't welcome?

Dr. Booker: I got the position because my husband was on the faculty. I was appointed to this nontenure track. I was given the opportunity to be an independent principal investigator and take graduate students, but I was not given the opportunity to be an assistant professor—and I didn't ask because it didn't seem like a reasonable thing to do. Some of the professors expressed the view that their arms had been twisted into giving me PI status because if I had left, my husband would have left. So that would tend to create the impression, one wasn't particularly welcome [laugh]. During the third year you can turn [the position] into an assistant professorship, and when that time came, although I had an NIH grant and had graduate students and was starting to publish papers, and I was significantly better than the male assistant professor who had been hired the year I was hired, I was told that I was not going to be made an assistant professor. Toward the end of my fifth year or so, I learned through somebody—I didn't even know this—that you can't stay at the university beyond a certain point if you're not tenured. At that point I began to worry and feel angry because I was, in my view, doing pretty well and getting invited places—to lecture.

It was clear that I had a lower status. And I had the smallest office in the department, and I had outgrown my lab space. I wouldn't have been able to do research that I was doing if my husband didn't give me lab space. So there was a long list of reasons why I didn't feel like I belonged. It was not a very pleasant experience. Having said that, I'm grateful to them for making me a PI (and not all universities will do that, they're very protective of that status, for reasons that aren't clear to me because I think the more PIs the better). They also did give me some lab space and some start-up sums, so although I expressed the view that they didn't treat me well, they gave me enough, and that made all the difference. But they didn't give me enough so that I was on the same playing field as everybody else. Over time that wears on you. And then after you start doing well, it wears on you more because you reach a point where you expect to be rewarded. "Wait, now I'm doing well. Now don't I get something for [laugh] all these sacrifices?" And the answer is "No." So moving was the only viable option, to go to a place where I would start out more or less equal and then see what happened.

Dr. Booker described other ways in which she had experienced active discrimination.

With regard to the department, I don't think there were high points. My group and my science were a constant source of pleasure. The third year review was a low-point when I realized it was looking like a dead-end position even though I was doing well. I wasn't that pleased when I found that I made $3,000 less than the assistant professor who had been hired when I was hired, even though I had more grants and more students and was also teaching—I was doing the full load of teaching—all of the work of the faculty. Just the sense that I couldn't get out of that position is a chronic thing that wears on you. If you dwell on the negative in your life, you're not going to get anywhere. So these are things I kept suppressed because there's really no point. . . . You might as well dwell on the things that make you happy. A chairman came in from outside, and I was promoted to tenure from a nontenure-track position because he took an active interest. If he had not appeared on the scene, it would not have happened. In life when so many things come down to chance, where it doesn't really matter how you do—that's not such a great thought. . . .

I think that happens to a lot of women: they're doing just a fine and dandy job supporting departments and teaching and raising money, and as long as they're willing to do that and their alternative is worse, then they're kept in those positions or kept at the level they are at, because what's the incentive?

Like Dr. Booker, other women reported that despite similar training and preparation for an academic career, they began their faculty appointments with fewer academic resources than men (e.g., protected time for research, laboratory space, and research assistance) (Tesch et al. 1995). Recent surveys continue to show lower salaries for women scientists, particularly at the senior levels, and even with new appointments of women (Ash et al. 2004; Zielinska 2008). Female physicians still earn only 82 percent of what male physicians earn, even after accounting for differences in numbers of hours worked, specialty, practice setting, and research productivity (Carr et al. 1993; Baker 1996; Ash et al. 2004; Murphy 2005). Dr. Carter, an early career faculty physician participating in our study, found out that she wasn't paid as much as other people at her level. It took over three months of negotiations with several levels of management to resolve her pay inequity. Then she reviewed the public salary records and saw that women in her institution in general were not paid as well as men. After she told other women about her raise, at least three others received salary increases. Dr. Carter asked, "Why were our salaries so much lower, and it took my getting this raise and telling others to get people's salaries up to where they should have been?" Her question still stands.

These facts set into relief the idealism and dedication of medical school faculty. Dr. Booker did remark that she was not pleased to be making less than a man with fewer credentials, but in general salary inequities were not a major complaint of our interviewees. Anyone who wanted a larger income would have left academic medicine, or not chosen it to begin with. They stayed because this was work they wanted to do. Dr. Haitham summed up her own experience:

I think there is a strong discrimination, gender based, ethnicity based. That always does depress you because—I've been fairly successful, and I think it's partially just a fluke— but I'm not sure how equal it could get, how they would fight the discrimination, which is very subtle. In the days when this must have been open discrimination, it probably wasn't easier because you knew what was happening. But I think at this stage it's all very subtle. It's hard to—whether it be gender or ethnicity—to reach the top even if you are ambitious enough.

Some of our interviewees reported experiences of sexual harassment by co-workers or superiors that not only made them feel even more like outsiders but led to their actually being ostracized. Most such incidents occurred during the training phase of their careers. One scientist reported that as a graduate student (getting her PhD), she had been sexually harassed and stalked on an ongoing basis by a technician in her lab. When she complained, first to her laboratory director and then to her department chair, neither took it seriously. Moreover, she was socially ostracized by the male students in her department "because they all took the technician's side; they all thought I was crazy." Eventually a court order was brought against the stalker.

Self-Doubt

A major effect of women's outsider status and the lack of recognition of their professional abilities is that they feel devalued and are chronically self-doubting. Peggy McIntosh, a scholar at the Wellesley College Stone Center for Women, notes that even highly accomplished women often say they feel like frauds who do not belong in the upper levels of social hierarchies of knowledge, authority, and power. McIntosh attributes this feeling to frequent, pervasive social messages that women (and "lower-caste or minority men") do not belong at the top of the hierarchy (McIntosh 1985). Thus, despite Professor Booker's success (and abundant evidence thereof, including national recognition for her scientific work), she still felt intellectually inferior to her male peers. She said she felt like an impostor, lacked full confidence in her own abilities, and described herself as "dumber" than men.

Dr. Booker: I've always had the sense that I have been successful in science because somehow I'm able to synthesize information in a way that leads to these creative flashes. But that I'm actually not that good when it comes to quantitative stuff. . . . My husband gets frustrated when I say this, but it's a pervasive feeling I've always had, which also is a reason I made the choices I made. If you are not good enough to do something, you really shouldn't try, because you are just going to make yourself unhappy. So when I'm around men, I have this chronic sense that maybe I'm dumber than they are. When I'm around women, I'm not burdened by that thought. I feel that we are more allies, whether we are or not. But I'm sure that relates to some psychological aspect of my upbringing that is not necessarily widely shared, but it's there. Definitely, there's a component of having grown up listening to [people saying] men are this and that and are smart, they're the geniuses.

McIntosh would connect this feeling of self-doubt, at least in part, to Dr. Booker's having internalized the assumption that as a woman she has no place as a public representative of status and power. The widespread nature of such self-doubt is evident in a comment made by Sonia Sotomayor, the newest United States Supreme Court Justice, who grew up in a housing project in the Bronx. "I have spent my years since Princeton, while at law school and in my various professional jobs, not feeling completely a part of the worlds I inhabit," she said, adding that despite her accomplishments, "I am always looking over my shoulder wondering if I measure up" (Zeleny 2009).

How Women Cope

Faculty members described various responses to the difficulties of their workplaces, ranging from "keeping their heads down" and doing the best they could to figuring out how to operate within the system while not losing their own perspective.

Keeping Quiet

Some women reacted to the inequities they perceived by deciding to keep quiet and just getting on with their work, trying not to attract attention and avoiding confrontation with authoritarian leaders. They inferred that this was the safer path and that they could accomplish their professional goals more effectively without directly confronting unfairness. Thus, Dr. Booker commented:

> I have noticed that it's better to get to be successful, or to do your work and keep your head down, than to draw attention to complaints that may be legitimate but aren't getting in the way of your accomplishments. It may make them harder. If you don't have a big enough lab space, you have to walk over two buildings to do an experiment. It's inconvenient, because you're rolling a cart back and forth, and you're doing these things that nobody else has to do. It makes it harder, but it doesn't make it impossible. It doesn't prevent you from doing it. It just means that you don't have what other people have.

> Dr. Carter: It was so stressful to participate and risk what I didn't want to risk—it's not that I kept my mouth shut 100 percent, but I didn't, for example, bring up difficult questions at faculty meetings. . . . There were people in our department who lost their jobs over their being expressive. Their lives were made absolutely miserable. There was no question about that and it was even investigated at one point by the dean. It was pretty bad.

Creating "Microenvironments"

Instead of trying to upend the entire system, some highly successful women created their own microenvironments within the medical school in which they built the kind of collegial relationships and work ethos that they considered appropriate for carrying out their work to their own high standards. They talked about being successful and effective as leaders by focusing on the interpersonal manner in which the work was done. The same themes of creating work groups where people got to know each other well and developed trust emerged in all areas: the research laboratory, education, and clinical departments. For example, like Dr. Booker, Dr. Haitham created a secure environment for herself and her research group. Dr. Anderson, an internist, created a supportive microculture in a clinical setting.

Dr. Haitham: I wanted to create and control my own environment so I didn't have to put up with doing things I think are unethical and lack integrity. It actually worked very well. I had a small group for a while and I just ran the little group. And then things started getting a little more successful and gradually the group kept growing. And then there came this rather big success, and it all happened almost really with no planning.

Dr. Anderson: As we were trying to build this department, recruiting new people, etc., we've tried to change the atmosphere, and we've tried to make it supportive . . . someone has clinic that's about to start but they're having difficulty with certain procedures . . . I'll do the procedures and you go to clinic. You don't need to be stressed about it. We will work together. And so after that happened, then another faculty would do it for me. I like doing what I'm doing. I like the little environment that we've been able to create. That is very satisfying.

Addressing the Work-Centric Culture

Some women explicitly rejected the conventional work-centric, all-consuming medical school culture by making a deliberate effort to create balance in their own lives. These women wanted to have successful careers on their own terms.

Dr. Harwood: I made some conscious decisions early on about finding little ways to make the department not the center of my universe, not having it eat my life . . . I realized I was going to need a physical outlet . . . that really got me out of the intellectual realm . . . I needed to build balance into my life, otherwise I'd make myself crazy. . . . You really can do it in a fifty- to sixty-hour week . . . and your productivity doesn't suffer. That was one mentality, the whole macho science mentality . . . eighteen hours a day in the lab crap.

Dr. Jones: I like to pursue interests like dance or gardening or cooking or having friends. Those things are important to me . . . it becomes hard to do that because of a need to devote so much time to the career. That's always been [my goal] . . . giving me the feeling that I've got one foot in and one foot out of academic medicine. . . . I'll stay as long as it's meaning[ful]. . . . I can do it on my own terms.

Being a "Tempered Radical"

Many women faculty in academic medicine appear to be what Meyerson and Scully call "tempered radicals." They coined this term to describe individuals—generally women or members of underrepresented minority groups—who identify with their organizations and want to succeed within them but are also committed to a cause, community, or set of ideas that are different from, or in conflict with, the organization's dominant culture. Thus, they have a goal to create change within the organization, but they go about it in a moderate, "tempered" way, working from within. The word tempered also takes on a second meaning in this context: that these women are strengthened, as metal is tempered, through the experience of operating in such challenging environments.

When outsiders express opinions intemperately, they are likely to alienate those in power and threaten their professional identity. Tempered radicals have learned to recognize this vulnerability and therefore to "play the game" in order to get ahead, while they avoid becoming fully co-opted. In this way they preserve their personal identity, values and beliefs, while biding their time until they achieve the credibility and position that will allow them to effect change. In tempered radicals, both personal and professional identities are strong. However, the disconnect between the two may engender feelings of ambivalence, guilt, and self-doubt. Often, they feel they must keep their nontraditional feelings and opinions to themselves for fear of undermining their own credibility or even to avoid retaliation or punishment. As a result they often feel lonely and isolated.

Like Meyerson and Scully's tempered radicals, our interviewees were simultaneously trying to master the "norms" of the profession in order to advance professionally while recognizing that these same norms might perpetuate systemic inequity. They developed dual identities: they were successful within medical school culture and fully understood the norms of behavior and what it took to succeed, but at the same time they maintained an outsider's perspective. However, the values and beliefs of their professional/organizational identity conflicted with the values and beliefs of their personal/extra-organizational identity.

Dr. Rosenberg: I think what became clear to me is the university's interest was in power and money, not in improving medical care or intellectual growth. I got high up enough in the organization so that I could actually see that quite clearly. I was on the leadership committee of the medical center. It was all money and power, and that was for me extremely disillusioning. So I felt increasingly a sense of nonbelonging to the university community.

Like the tempered radicals described by Meyerson and Scully, some medical faculty used their power and understanding to stand up for others. Dr. Rossi, a basic scientist early in her career, and Dr. Ireland, a leading physician, both showed this strength:

Dr. Rossi: The fact that there are no women here keeps me staying here because I feel [that] I have to make a stance and show the younger generation that there are women here. It's tough.

Dr. Ireland: I can use the privilege that I have now . . . to get things done for other people. I'm in the midst of one of those discussions right now in which I don't think a chair is treating a faculty member very well, and I'm tempering it to not push his buttons too much. But I do believe the power of my position and the power of my experience will get it worked out okay for the faculty member.

Some of our interviewees made it clear that they understood how to play the game in order to accomplish objectives of their own. Dr. Tonder, for example, explained that it was necessary to lie low for a long time to get to a position where one could have an influence:

Dr. Tonder: One of the errors women make is that we don't understand that you need to aspire to certain roles to get authority. I wanted to make change, and I was naïve enough not to understand that the first thing I needed to do was get the power. I thought I could just convince people to do the things they needed to do on the power of the ideas and by lining up political support. And I found that, particularly as a woman, until you got way, way, way, way, way at the top, much higher than a man would need to get to get the same thing accomplished, you were wise to just keep your nose clean. . . . To get into a position of power or leadership, women need to be more savvy about how to manipulate in a group environment than I was, a less direct approach, perhaps, a willingness to be there from the very first thing in the morning till the very end of the night. Put in more hours than almost anybody else so that people saw you as one of the boys and that meant showing up—traveling to meetings that you don't really need to go to because that's where they're all going to be. People who bring in grant money, who don't rock the boat too much especially early on, [who] spend the first ten years or so doing their research, bringing in grants, publishing and not threatening anybody's fiefdom. People who are willing to come in very early and stay very late and do whatever assignment they're given without trying to go back and say, would it be smarter if we did it this way?

The intransigence of the difficulties women describe in this chapter is sobering. However there is hope that these "outsiders within" will—sooner rather than later—be able to combine the knowledge and thoughts of the insider with the critical attitude of the outsider, questioning the validity of the status quo and developing new bodies of knowledge beyond existing paradigms. Therein lies a real benefit that women, as well as other underrepresented groups, can bring to the medical school system and to health care generally. Some of the women leaders described in the next chapter are in fact examples of tempered radicals who are already making changes in academic medical centers. They have moved beyond feeling that they must bide their time because equality can be achieved only in incremental steps. They, like our own C - Change partnership of medical schools, are attempting to drive change more rapidly.

REFERENCES

Acker J. Hierarchies, jobs, bodies: a theory of gendered organizations. Gender Society. 1990;4(2):139–58.

Ash AS, Carr PL, Goldstein R, Friedman RH. Compensation and advancement of women in academic medicine: is there equity? Ann Intern Med. 2004;141:205–12.

Baker L. Differences in earnings between male and female physicians. N Engl J Med. 1996;334:960–4.

Biernat M, Fuegen K. Shifting standards and the evaluation of competence: complexity in gender-based judgment and decision making. J Social Issues. 2001; 57:707–24.

Carnes M, Geller S, Fine E, Sheridan J, Handelsman J. NIH director's pioneer awards: could the selection process be biased against women? J Womens Health. 2005;14(8):684–91.

Carr PL, Ash AS, Friedman RH, Scaramucchi A, Barnett R, Szalacha L, Palepu A, Moskowitz M. Faculty perceptions of gender discrimination and sexual harassment in academic medicine. Ann Intern Med. 2000;132:889–96.

Carr P, Freidman R, Moskowitz M, Kazis L. Comparing the status of women and men in academic medicine. Ann Intern Med. 1993;119:908–13.

Carr PL, Szalacha L, Barnett R, Caswell C, Inui T. A ton of feathers: gender discrimination in academic medical careers and how to manage it. J Womens Health. 2003;12(10):1009–18.

Costrich N, Feinstein J, Kidder L, Marecek J, Pascale L. When stereotypes hurt: three studies of penalties for sex-role reversals. J Exp Soc Psychol. 1975;11:520–30.

Dreifus C. Conversation with Carol W. Greider on winning a Nobel prize. New York Times, October 13, 2009.

Eagly A. Sex differences in social behavior: a social-role interpretation. Hillsdale, NJ: Erlbaum; 1987.

Eagly A, Carli L. Through the labyrinth: the truth about how women become leaders. Boston: Harvard Business School Press; 2007.

Ely RJ, Meyerson DE. Theories of gender in organizations: a new approach to organizational analysis and change. Res Organiz Behav. 2000;22:103–51.

Heilman ME. Description and prescription: how gender stereotypes prevent women's ascent up the organizational ladder. J Social Issues. 2001;57(4):657–74.

Heilman ME, Wallen AS, Fuchs D, Tamkins MM. Penalties for success: reactions to women who succeed at male gender-type tasks. J Appl Psychol. 2004;89:416–27.

Hyde S, Mertz J. Gender, culture and mathematics performance. Proc Natl Acad Sci USA. 2009;106:8801–7.

Jagsi R, Tarbell NJ, Henailt LE. The representation of women on the editorial boards of major medical journals: a 35-year perspective [letter]. Arch Intern Med. 2008;168:544–8.

Keiser J, Utzinger J, Singer B. Gender composition of editorial boards of general medical journals. Lancet. 2003;362:1336.

LaFrance M. Gender and interruptions: individual infraction or violation of social order? Psychol Women Q. 1992;16:497–512.

Leahey E, Guo G. Gender differences in mathematical trajectories. Social Forces. 2001;80(2):713–32.

Ley TJ, Hamilton BH. The gender gap in NIH grant applications. Science. 2008; 322:1472–4.

Mansfield HC. Manliness. New Haven, CT: Yale University Press; 2006.

McIntosh P. Feeling like a fraud. Wellesley, MA: Wellesley Centers for Women; 1985.

Murphy E. Getting even: why women don't get paid like men—and what to do about it. New York: Touchstone; 2005.

Rudman LA. Self-promotion as a risk factor for women: the costs and benefits of counterstereotypical impression management. J Pers Soc Psychol. 1998;74(3): 629–45.

Scheman N. Engenderings: constructions of knowledge, authority, and privilege. New York: Routledge; 1993.

Steinpreis RE, Anders KA, Ritzke D. The impact of gender on the review of the curricula vitae of job applicants and tenure candidates: a national empirical study. Sex Roles. 1999;41:509–28.

Tesch BJ, Wood HM, Helwig AL, Nattinger AB. Promotion of women physicians in academic medicine. Glass ceiling or sticky floor? JAMA. 1995;273(13):1022–5.

Trix F, Penska C. Exploring the color of glass: letters of recommendation for female and male medical faculty. Discourse Society. 2003;14:191–220.

Uhlmann EL, Cohen GL. Constructed criteria: redefining merit to justify discrimination. Psychol Sci. 2005;16:474–80.

Valian V. Why so slow? The advancement of women. Cambridge, MA: MIT Press; 1998.

Wenneras C, Wold A. Nepotism and sexism in peer-review. Nature. 1997;387: 341–3.

Zeleny J. Obama chooses Sotomayor for Supreme Court nominee. New York Times. May 26, 2009. Available at: http://thecaucus.blogs.nytimes.com/2009/05/26/obama-makes-decision-on-supreme-court-nominee/.

Zielinska E. The scientist 2008 life science salary survey. Scientist. 2008;22:45.

chapter 7

Women as Leaders

> I turn now to our shared vocation of leadership in the world of action. This may seem more like a leap than a turn, but none of the great wisdom traditions would look upon this segue with surprise. Go far enough on the inner journey, they all tell us—go past ego toward true self—and you end up not lost in narcissism but returning to the world, bearing more gracefully the responsibilities that come with being human. A leader is someone with the power to project either shadow or light upon some part of the world, and upon the lives of the people who dwell there. —Parker Palmer (1999)

Even though substantial numbers of women have been graduating from medical schools for many years, they continue to occupy far fewer of the higher decision-making positions than one would expect from their representation within the profession. To understand better the source of this discrepancy, I turn again to the women interviewed who had achieved seniority and were in leadership positions. This chapter summarizes their perspectives and experiences, as well as the views of other women aspiring to contribute maximally in their fields.

Almost all the women leaders were married and mothers. They came from all domains of academic medicine: patient care, research, medical education, and administration. Their comments reflect their fine personal qualities and their ability to be superior leaders. The stories they tell shine a light on the past and present culture of academic medicine and also suggest ways that power can be used more constructively in medical schools.

It is troubling that both the popular and academic press perpetuate a widespread assumption that women do not want to assume leadership roles. We did not find this to be true in medicine. When asked about leadership, female—as well as male—interviewees talked of being energized and fulfilled as leaders. Nor did the women lack ambition. As Dr. Rouge explained,

> There is no shortage of ambition among the women I work with; anybody who says that women's advancement has fallen behind because women have no interest is a hundred percent wrong. That's not what I see.

Rosabeth Moss Kanter explored the notion that women have more limited aspirations than men and concluded that both men and women limit their aspirations, decrease their work commitment, and sometimes dream of escape if they decide that their progress is blocked (Kanter 1977). It could well be that women's aspirations are limited by a lack of role models and of opportunities to become leaders. As we will see, when such an opportunity is available, they eagerly accept it.

What we did find in our own study was that women related to leadership in a manner that did not wholly conform with perspectives on leading expressed by the male leaders we interviewed. It was quite rare for women to state, "I want to be a leader"; men were more likely to say that they sought leadership positions or that they should be leaders. Men reported constantly being urged into leadership, or of being directly asked to lead, and then described the satisfaction of being successful in those roles. Another difference was that women rarely favored the authoritarian or "power-over" model commonly associated with traditional leadership in our culture. Their enthusiasm for leadership lay in the desire to advance ideas or to make meaningful improvements.

Nonetheless, regardless of their ambitions, our data show that women faced both external and internal barriers to leadership, growing both out of others' reactions to the idea of women in positions of authority and from women's own negative response to the behavior they saw current leaders in their institutions practicing themselves or rewarding in others.

Barriers to Women Becoming Leaders

There is a dearth of women leaders not only in academic medicine but in all professional sectors of the economy. In 2001, 47 percent of workers were women, but in Fortune 500 companies, women were seldom present in the boardroom; only 0.4 percent of CEOs and only 3 percent of the highest paid corporate officers were female. Currently, only 17 percent of U.S. Senators and 17 percent of Congress members are women. Although about 30 percent of lawyers are women, women constitute only 15 percent of law firm partners and 5 percent of managing partners in large firms (Catalyst 2000). The lack of women leaders in academic medicine, therefore, seems to be a reflection of barriers to women's leadership that are present in our society generally.

Nonconscious Bias

Research in a variety of occupational fields indicates that women in leadership roles—especially in male dominated occupations—face nonconscious or implicit resistance to their holding such jobs. There is a robust literature describing how female leaders receive less favorable evaluations than their male counterparts in male-dominated occupations and how women are penalized in leadership roles (Eagly et al. 1992; Eagly and Karau 2002). As noted in Chapter 6, women are judged to be less competent than men whose performance is identical. For example, Heilman asked fifty men and fifty women to evaluate a woman candidate for a managerial position. She found that when women represented less than 25 percent of the applicant pool, they were evaluated less favorably by both men and women. Virginia Schein reviewed studies on bias against female leaders in the United States, United Kingdom, Germany, China, and Japan and found that in all these countries, men were perceived to be more qualified as managers than women (Schein 2001). In academic medicine, women constitute far fewer than 25 percent of the applicant pool for almost all leadership positions. It is the rare medical school that takes the trouble to educate the members of search committees about nonconscious bias in the evaluation and selection process, although some male leaders are starting to stipulate that at least one woman candidate must be interviewed for leadership positions.

In another series of experiments by Heilman, participants evaluated the likability of male and female employees in "male-type" jobs and "female-type" jobs. She found that there was no difference in the ratings of competence between female and male employees when the prior success of the person being assessed was made explicit. However, when information about performance was ambiguous, successful female employees were rated significantly less competent than successful male employees. Successful female employees were also liked significantly less than male employees when there was clear evidence of success. Heilman also found that successful female employees were significantly less likable than equally successful male employees in male-type jobs, but significantly more likable in female-type jobs. There was a clear tendency for women in male-type jobs to be characterized as more interpersonally hostile than men in the same type jobs. In a third study, Heilman used male and female employees in a financial services company to assess the effect of likability on evaluation and on rewards given to employees. She found that likable employees were evaluated more favorably and recommended more highly for salary increases and promotion than less likable employees, regardless of gender. Notably, both women and men evaluators exhibited these biases (Heilman 2001). Our research provides many examples of biases limiting women's advancement in academic medical centers.

Nonconscious bias that penalizes women leaders suggests another reason why women do not put themselves forward to become leaders. It seems likely that women have been conditioned to protect themselves against the effects of this bias through a nonconscious reluctance to be seen as assertively seeking leadership and power or as emulating male leaders. This lack of self-assertion has then been misconstrued to mean that women actually do not want to be leaders. As mentioned previously, C - Change medical school survey data show no statistical difference in women's and men's aspirations for leadership.

Conscious Resistance

Another significant barrier to women becoming leaders is that they encounter a great deal of quite conscious resistance at the highest echelons of academic medicine. A number of women leaders who did make it described this resistance. When Dr. Goldsmith sought to become a department chair, she discovered that it was extremely difficult to be considered for that position because it was so unusual for a woman to chair a medical school department.

> Dr. Goldsmith: I was looking at a chair job at another institution. The
> dean actually called me up and told me he couldn't offer me the job be-

cause I was a woman, because "they'd never had a woman chair before," and he "just couldn't do it." That's probably the most blunt example. He ended up writing a very nice letter to tell them to hire me here, when I applied for this position, but that he couldn't do it himself.

But even after Dr. Goldsmith assumed the chair position at the second university, she faced overt resistance. She had believed that colleagues and supervisors would look out for and support a new person in a leadership role and was surprised to find not only that she received no support, but that some were determined to oust her from the position.

> Dr. Goldsmith: Chairs here have always been men, and the man who was stepping down actually was trying to orchestrate giving this job to his protégé who had been here training under him his whole career. The search committee here actually decided they wanted a change, and in doing so, tried to look at outside candidates. I came and looked at the job and realized the place was ready for a change.
>
> But when I took the job it was shocking. Everyone had figured they would give it to the inside candidate anyway. Probably the most shocked person was the previous chair. The person [who] didn't get the job—he's still angry about it. He still can't talk to me. Because many of the faculty really loved him and many of the faculty thought he was going to get it. Many people thought I would come here, [but] there was no way I could make it. That I would be out the door in months, if not a year or two. But, of course, that didn't happen. I came and decided this was going to work, and I had lots of things to offer. I think now there is no question that it's a better department since I came; we've hired about twenty-four people; clinical activity and research activity are up, so it's been fine. But it definitely was a shock to the whole surgical system that I got the job.

People had actually laid bets that she would not last.

> Dr. Goldsmith: A lot of people didn't think they would ever take a woman surgeon to run [the department], and so probably the most successful thing is that I've lasted two years. And actually people will tell you, we are successful here. Whereas I think a lot of people had money bet on the opposite—that it would never work out. [laughing]

Others from Dr. Goldsmith's institution reported that the surgical residents in her department wrote her a group letter telling her that they did not welcome her. Since then, Dr. Goldsmith has increased the proportion of female surgical residents and improved the clinical enterprise and research efforts.

Many women perceived as a barrier their own intention to bring about change, because of the resistance of current leaders:

> Dr. Tonder: A lot of people were very supportive of the new ideas, but the people who were in the positions to get in the way, the chairman of the department and his associate chairman, the dean of the medical school, these were people for whom such change was always greeted with a great deal of anxiety.

Another woman leader who subsequently left her medical school described an authoritarian, narcissistic long-standing chief who had created an environment where faculty feared supporting someone out of favor with him. Any change had the potential of undermining the leader's control and was consequently stopped.

> Dr. Frank: This individual could not bear anybody else being in the limelight. He was just so narcissistic that that was enormously threatening to him. He could have had every benefit from my efforts, but he couldn't risk that. I don't think he was very aware; he'd been there a long time. There was no boundary between his own identity and the role he had in the school. He just saw my success as enormously threatening; he really didn't want anybody to come in and make any change, unless he did it. So he was very malicious in the way he undermined our work. And I was very naïve. I didn't recognize the situation for what it was, until too late. He had built such a culture of fear in that place. . . . People had seen him behave in this way many times before. So they knew all the signs.

As we saw in Chapter 5, Dr. Venetia believed that current leaders in her institution deliberately installed weak education leaders to decrease competition with the clinical enterprise. In the same way, Dr. Harwood thought that her leadership appointed only weak female leaders, so as not to threaten the existing male-dominated power structure.

Dr. Harwood: The women in leadership were—I've come to believe—chosen because they were weak. No strong woman leaders in the medical school. I think it's to their advantage not to have strong female leaders: ". . . they're "troublesome". . . . "they have ideas."

Some faculty attributed the absence of women in positions of authority to inattention rather than intent. For example, Dr. Booker commented:

I think part of the reason for lack of progress [regarding women] relates to the fact that there aren't . . . many people with real power who take a personal interest in the issue of women's leadership. Not that they're actively opposed, but they have other things on their mind; and they're not personally standing in someone's way, they're just not helping, so nothing happens.

Another way of preventing women from advancing (maybe inadvertently) was to put them on too many committees; assign teaching duties; or give them extra students to advise. These responsibilities could occupy a great deal of time, detracting from time available for research or other scholarship. Committee work contributes far less than other types of duties to promotion or other advancement.

Dr. Tonder: I ended up being the only woman repeatedly on committee after committee after committee after committee, because I had to be. I was the only [one in my position] who was a woman in the medical school in the clinical side.

Dr. Risen: I got put on a lot of committees where they needed a junior person or a female. And I didn't get protected as much as I should have from committee work. . . . Around here, when you need somebody to teach or you've got a kid [student] with a problem, I think they tend to send you to a junior female. . . . They just dumped them on me. They said, "She can take care of them." . . . They knew that I wouldn't let those students flounder.

This "dumping" is also another example of devaluing the nurturing of others, which we saw in Chapter 6.

Fear of Compromising Integrity

Research indicates that even though, as youngsters, women have grand goals and clear ambitions, as adults many associate ambition with self-aggrandizement, egotism, and manipulation (Fels 2004). Certainly a strong theme that emerged in our interviews was that women were often reluctant to assume leadership positions because they believed they would have to compromise their own values in such positions and did not want to risk losing their integrity. Because of the nature of medical school culture, women often assumed that becoming a leader meant self-aggrandizement and the transactional use of power to confer or withhold rewards or benefits or to penalize. Women felt a moral distress because their own values were so out of sync with what they saw played out in their institutions. Almost all the women leaders we interviewed, but fewer of the male leaders, said they felt that their own values were not aligned with institutional values. This difference conforms to our finding (reported in Chapter 5) that women were more disturbed than men by the difference between their own values and those of their institutions.

Women described different ways of avoiding such a values conflict: changing their duties, leaving the organization, or not applying for leadership positions. A successful leader said,

> Dr. Westenfelder: At the few times when I felt there was a values conflict, I've negotiated a change of duties so that I didn't have to have a personal values conflict. One of the things I learned from my old dean is that it is important to understand your values as a hierarchy and that you can't serve all of them all the time, but you need to know which ones are key, which are the values you must serve all the time in order to feel true to yourself.

Dr. Jones described poignantly her distress over the unethical and disrespectful behavior of the leaders she knew and concluded sadly that she did not want to be a leader, because she feared she might have to behave in ways she considered shameful.

> You look to leadership to set the tone—whether this is a place where people are heard and respected. There have been times when leadership in

my institution appeared to have its own agenda. It didn't value the things that I valued. For instance, it didn't value diversity, or the experiences of women, or the voices of women. It didn't value clinicians. Women's issues are very important to me, but if it never gets brought up or never gets heard, . . . women become invisible; if that is an environment the leadership allows, it becomes unattractive to me.

Like the leader I saw in my early career. There's no way I want to be in a situation where I have to be deceitful in order to get people to do what they need to do . . . or have to work on scheming and cover-ups as a way of doing my job. That's what I think he felt he must have had to do, hide money . . . or at least to cook the books a little bit . . . and then not be concerned about a student's career, a fellow's career, because one had financial obligations to meet. That was what leadership looked like to me. . . . It was not something I ever wanted to do.

Dr. Geordino expressed similar sentiments.

In the dean's strategic planning meetings I was just a fly on the wall trying to learn, and did I learn!!! I learned that I didn't want to be a big dean, no matter what. At least, until the principles and the values of the way academic medicine is managed change dramatically.

She had begun attending these meetings after she told the dean she was interested in a leadership position. What was evident in those meetings was a lack of respect for individual faculty.

Dr. Geordino: At one point I thought I was interested in being associate dean for academic affairs or student affairs. The dean, very supportive of women and very helpful, had me attend his strategic planning meeting, a group that most faculty don't know exists. It's basically the dean's closest advisors, the finance officers, the academic deans, and the chairs of the two largest departments, surgery and internal medicine. I was the only woman in those meetings. I was treated as a child by at least one of the department chairs. He would shake his finger at me, [as if] I were a small child. And the things they were discussing at that meeting were fascinating and disturbing. People's lives were talked about very casually, their lives and careers. I learned things that I'd just as soon not know. And I thought that though individually the deans are folks with high values and principles, when it came down to the business of running the school, it was more just business. The attitude was "no margin, no mission." People's entire lives or careers might be just, "Well we can't let him or her do that . . . no, we don't care if they go someplace else." I found this very disturbing and decided that I really didn't want to be a part of that. I'd rather continue in the advocacy type role I have now. I don't want to feel that I have to compromise my principles in a position. I don't think I could fit in one of those [leadership] roles and be successful—they probably wouldn't keep me there [laugh], because of the way I would handle things.

Dr. Geordino linked the short tenure of the few women who did attain leadership positions to their unwillingness to compromise their values, which led to their being forced out or leaving voluntarily. In her view, male leaders were more willing to adapt their values to the work at hand.

Not that the men we know and work with don't have values and prin-ciples; they apply them differently to their work. [After discussing this with colleagues] we think that's one of the major reasons that women we've seen be successful for a short period of time leave or are forced out of the institution.

It is important to note that women rarely spoke of their mothering or family care responsibilities as barriers to seeking promotion. When they did, they explained that their advancement had been held back because they limited their travel and the number of hours they worked each week because of family obligations. These women were deeply involved with their families but also wanted rich, meaningful, and rewarding profes-sional lives; they did not experience a conflict between the two.

Overall, no single factor can be identified that prevents women from becoming leaders. Instead, there seems to be a cumulative effect resulting from all the causes described above: nonconscious bias, conscious resis-tance to change, especially when introduced by someone with an outsider perspective, women's distrust and distaste regarding the people in charge, and, significantly, the belief that taking a leadership position necessarily meant compromising one's integrity. These feelings constituted one of the most disturbing results of our study. They colored women's aspirations and—although certainly a testament to their character—became a barrier to women's advancing in their careers. This quite significant reason for women's failure to advance has not previously received attention. But as we will see, these beliefs were inaccurate, for other forms of leadership are possible.

Women's Paths to Leadership

Women tended not to seek power for its own sake or for the trappings power is associated with. Their justifications for taking a leadership position were based on the assumption that authority or power could be honorably held only if it were clearly related not to individual gain but to service to others. Some women, speaking about this instinctive modesty, explained that they had had to grow into positions of authority:

> Dr. Venetia: I tend to have a self-effacing personality. It is uncomfortable for me sometimes to take on a leadership role, if it means being in the spotlight. But if it is about advancing ideas and principles, and not about me as an individual . . . then, I can justify doing it.

Dr. Venetia continued:

> Initially, I would have said "No," but you get to a point in your career where you realize that people are looking up to you, and you think, "Oh, I guess I have something important to say," and suddenly you feel it would be nice to be considered a leader. It's a way of serving. It's almost like the servant-leader concept. It's like an obligation: you should do it; you shouldn't hold back.

Other women came to leadership positions "accidentally," as described by Drs. Haitham and Risen, both basic scientists in leadership positions, or because they were encouraged by their families of origin, like Dr. Westenfelder, or simply accepted positions that were offered. It is likely, though, that their success was mostly the result of their talent, hard work, and aspirations; as Pasteur noted, "chance favors those with a prepared mind."

Dr. Haitham: I never had a plan of what I wanted to do. And most certainly I never had a plan to be successful in this business, successful as measured by positions and titles and all that. What I really thought I would do when I came here was to work in a lab, somebody else's lab, and just enjoy the [science] . . . So leadership and being where I am now was never part of the plan. I think it was totally accidental.

Dr. Risen: I've never thought I wanted it [leadership], but when I see somebody else doing a really shitty job, like the guy who had this job before me . . . When they offered it to me, I said, "Yes. I'll take it; I'll fix that." So I guess maybe I did want it. I would never have said, "Give me that job." But when somebody said, "Dr. Risen, you could do this," at first, it scared me a little bit. I thought about it for a couple of days and I said, "You're right. I could do that." So I'm never a person who puts myself forward, but if someone gives it to me, I'll do it.

Dr. Westenfelder: And leadership had always been important to me. Not so much that I have sought it as that my family cultivated in me the notion of being able to assume it when you are asked to. I've had several national leadership positions too, and those all for me have been personal advancement. . . . I wasn't pursuing leadership, but I was ready to accept it. And I do think of myself as a leader with a small "L" anyway. Not in terms of position, but I think—this is going to sound immodest—that leadership is one of my gifts, and it's my responsibility to use that gift.

A number of women saw leadership as a path to getting things done and being able to do the work that was most meaningful to them while maintaining their integrity and the ethical standards they required of themselves. Some decided to actively seek leadership when they realized they could do a better job than their supervisors. This was the case with Dr. Frederick:

I never set out and said I wanted to be chief, or chair, or dean, or anything like that. I always sought such a position when I felt that the person above me wasn't doing as good a job as I thought I could and that affected adversely my work. It was more a feeling of what I wanted to do and how I wanted to do it.

From her early years as a trainee, Dr. Goldsmith wanted to make a difference and change the status quo but recognized that these could only be done by someone with power.

> Dr. Goldsmith: Being an intern or young faculty, you can complain, but no change is going to happen till you're in charge. As a resident, when things happened that I didn't like, I remember thinking, "You can't change any of this unless you're at the top." I'm not sure I ever thought, "Well, then, YOU need to go be in charge." But somewhere deep inside, I must have been thinking, "Just keep going and eventually you'll be able to change it, because you will be in charge." But I don't think it was a conscious thought at the time. . . .
>
> In my first two jobs, I was a very busy researcher, then I turned into more of a busy clinician, and then switched into being an administrator and visionary-type person. I felt successful in all those arenas. I'm not sure I ever thought about wanting leadership. I've had a very reactive career. For sure I never started off in medicine [wanting] to run a department of surgery. I don't think I even wanted to be a division chief. I think I wanted to be a surgeon because I loved the technical aspects and exciting part of it. I wanted to be a really good doctor, and I liked the academic part because of the ability to teach and also to do research.
>
> When I was younger, I didn't have numerous leadership positions; I wasn't a president or any of that. I would take positions that I liked in organizations, that I thought were the more fun positions; that was most important. I actually had a couple of mentors tell me that I would be good at leading groups. As I got older, I got to lead lots of groups as it was a very small medical center, and I think that's when I was first told by others that this was something I could do. I never sat saying "I want to be a chair," like some of my residents, mainly male, will come and say, "I want to be a Chair of Surgery. I want your job someday." I think it was more reaction to opportunity. And also realizing I probably wanted to make a difference and change surgery. In order for surgery to attract women and to be better, [it] was going to have to change. And it's about time for everybody that it changes.

A few women such as Dr. Rigoni, an internist early in her career, and Dr. Westenfelder did deliberately aim for decision-making positions.

Dr. Rigoni: On a good day, when I think things are going well, yes, I want to do academic medicine forever, and I feel great about this. I think if I set a great goal for myself, I'd love to be a division chief somewhere, someday. You need to set your expectations high in order to achieve great things.

Dr. Westenfelder: I saw very quickly that it was the leaders [who] changed the environment, and if you were not a leader, you were unable to make significant changes in how you lived and how you worked and how is your work environment. For me, that was the most important aspect—I really wanted to see more flexibility in the workforce. I wanted to have more diversity in the department. I wanted changes in the way patients were treated and the only way of getting to that was to become a leader.

Women's Goals as Leaders

To almost all the women we interviewed, leadership meant much more than being in charge. Many said they wanted to change the status quo by enriching their work environment with different perspectives. They saw women as being able to bring different qualities to decision making. An example of the style in which some approached their responsibilities is this comment from Dr. Mere, a department chair.

> One of the best trainings or the most important training I had that helped me as chair was that I was a mother . . . And I feel that kind of connection to my faculty, that I really want for them to be successful—and that they feel not only successful but they are enjoying their work—and they feel that they belong and that they have a voice in what happens to them.

In essence, these leaders were interested not in having power over others but in empowering their subordinates. Dr. Francesco contrasted "self-aggrandizing power" that constantly pulled inward, toward itself, to "centrifugal" power, which she described as "a dispersing power, an empowering of people in the environment." Dr. Westenfelder, an outstanding woman who had held a top position in a medical school and at the time of the interview was a national figure, said:

> I think the biggest challenge for women in medicine is to try to understand what it is that they could offer to academic medicine and to the

health care system. If women come into leadership positions but behave in conformity with the existing culture—which is a white male culture—it isn't bad, but it's incomplete, and there's no point in having women in power. The point is to bring different perspectives that can make things better for more people.

Dr. Goldsmith remarked,

> I don't think advancement is just garnering positions of power. Leading a group, being division chief, president of societies, chair of departments, not only obtaining these posts, but doing something with them. Making changes, making it better. I actually tell people the way I look at success is you showed up, you did a good job, and they would like you to come back because of what you did.

Changing Practices

A strong recurring theme was that changing standard medical school practices such as how medical students were trained or how patient care was delivered was an important reason for becoming a leader. Dr. Tonder, whose focus was education, felt passionately the need to change medical education, not simply to seek a title.

> It wasn't so much "position" that I wanted—I wanted to be able to ef-fect change. I didn't particularly care whether I was a chairman or a dean. I was offered an associate deanship, but the problem was that it was offered with no budgetary authority, and I didn't care about titles, I cared about being a change agent. . . .
>
> Did I want to be a dean of a medical school? No. It just never oc-curred to me. What I wanted was leadership of action, not leadership by power. If power was required to change something, then I was happy to accept the power to do it, but what I wanted to lead in was making change. I didn't want a deanship that was meaningless, just for the sake of having "Dean" in front of my name.

Dr. Peterson, a pediatrician, also became a leader through her desire to bring about paradigm shifts. Her comment below is reminiscent of the dual vision of the "tempered radicals" discussed in Chapter 6.

I didn't really think of myself as wanting to or needing to be in a leadership position earlier in my career. I wanted to contribute in some way to the field by shifting paradigms and ways of thinking about how to approach patients or how to address health issues in general in pediatrics. I realize that one of the ways you do that is by doing research. But then the way that you do research, as it turns out, is to continue the status quo with a different flavor. Doing research and trying to shift paradigms is not easy because you get up against people who say, "How is this relevant to what we've already been doing?" A lot of the medical literature is just rumination. It's repeating the same thing or moving an idea one step towards something else or just repackaging an idea.

I did a course related to patient interactions, and during that course, something shifted in my own understanding of how people are trained in medicine. One thing led to another, and now I'm at a point where I've studied the academic medical system in more detail and recognized that there is a desire to have a change but people are struggling because they have refined developing the status quo so much that they can't see how to change it. I've been a little eccentric over here, not buying into the status quo the way some of my contemporaries have. I actually am in a good position to contribute to the dialogue about how to change that. And that's where I say well, then it's up to me to decide if I'm going to pursue that in a leadership capacity as opposed to a follower [capacity].

For some, leadership meant the ability to improve the field of medicine on a broader scale. Dr. Harwood, a basic scientist, wanted to advance biomedical research through science policy.

I wanted to have a role in advancing biomedical research, not just be a laboratory scientist. Where I am now, doing science policy work and advocacy work for science, I think I have found the place I really wanted to be, acknowledged as a leader. I don't know if self-deprecating is the right word, but I tend to think of my role not really as a "leader" but a "facilitator." I want to be the one [who] gets all the right people together in the room and gives them the right question to answer, so that the answer will actually get us somewhere. If that's leadership, then yeah, I guess that's what I aspire to.

As we saw, Dr. Harwood described her role as a facilitator more than a leader, someone who gets the right people to work together. Dr. Harwood's and Dr. Frank's views on leadership are reminiscent of Ronald Heifetz's concepts when he describes leadership as mobilizing people in organizations to do "adaptive work." Rather than exercising authority and providing solutions, the leader does not need to have the answers but does create the structure or holding environment in which people can pay attention to tough problems and adapt to change themselves (Flower 1995; Heifetz and Linsky 2002).

Other women construed leadership positions differently, for example as heading up national committees. Dr. Knight, an obstetrician, commented:

> One of the national committees that I'm on—I would love to be the chair of that committee. Because I feel so strongly about these particular issues, I think that my being in the position of leadership there would help. I'm at a point in my career right now where I really want to do such good work.

Acting as Role Models

Many women leaders wanted to serve as role models for other women, since so few had had role models or mentors themselves. Dr. Cooper, a senior gynecologist/obstetrician, was one of several with this commitment.

> Dr. Cooper: I was very interested in women's health. Particularly, I was interested in becoming a leader myself because when I started out, there were no women in this field and there really were no women mentors for me, so I felt it was important that I should serve a role as a mentor for other women.

Dr. Haitham commented on her personal satisfaction in modeling integrity for her juniors.

> You can maintain your integrity, you can be kind, you can really take time to teach and still be successful in your own style. The highest compliment I've felt is when people who have left have said to me, "You taught me that integrity and success *can* go together."

Dr. Risen, a basic scientist in a leadership position, wanted to help her students as she had been helped.

> I like the academic environment. I like science as a career. I like helping students. I think that's probably the thing that's the most interesting to me. I like doing research. I like contributing to science. I don't think I ever wanted to be a powerful person. I don't think I'm interested in being a high profile person, but I like contributing. When I was a student, I never had an awful lot of confidence in myself. And a lot of people helped me along the way. And I think I wanted to do that for other students.

For Dr. Westenfelder, encouraging the next generation of leaders was her most important accomplishment.

> I firmly believe that the most meaningful thing I have done has been those times when I've been able to listen to and encourage upcoming leaders. The experiences in leadership have been a really important part of who I am as teacher and physician. It's another aspect related to healing. Those opportunities to influence and to help and encourage the next generation of leaders have been particularly energizing for me.

Characteristics of Women Leaders

It seems that women's leadership style frequently differs from that of men. Our own data agree with research in a range of occupational sectors that describes specific distinctions. Whereas traditionally, leadership was construed as a male pursuit, and leadership attributes were defined in stereotypically masculine language, more recently conceptual models describing effective leadership include a wider range of behaviors that have merged with stereotypical thinking about women. For example, building and sustaining teams, using emotional intelligence, and developing positive relationships have emerged as key attributes in the leadership effectiveness literature. Professors Alice Eagly and Linda Carli from Northwestern University and Wellesley College, and other colleagues who have conducted research in this area, have found that women leaders are more interpersonally oriented, more task-oriented, more democratic, and more transformational than men. It is true that there is a spectrum of leadership, in which some women use a more "male" style and some men a more "female" style, but over all, the pattern holds (Eagly and Johnson 1990; Eagly et al. 2003).

Relationship to power

As noted in Chapter 6, women's relationship to power tends to differ from men's. A leading gerontologist who subsequently left academic medicine (and labeled herself a "recovering academic") described how she came to realize that she used power differently from the predominant way she saw it used in her medical school.

> Dr. Violette: I remember distinctly the low point when I was making the decisions about whether this was the appropriate environment for me, distinctly thinking about power, and actually went and did some counseling. And came to the conclusion that the way I use power—I had always thought of myself as a powerful person in some ways, and yet it certainly didn't seem to be working well in that particular environment. The [counselor's] advice was that there are a lot of different ways of enacting power. I was not powerless; I just used power in a different way. I had wanted to be successful in that environment using power in my own way, and it really didn't work. Although the person thought I'd gotten along pretty far [laugh] even though I didn't know how to operate in that arena of power.

Dr. Violette believed in, and established, interdisciplinary teams to enhance clinical outcomes for patients. The members of such a team listen to the opinions of others whose position might be lower in the hierarchy; e.g., a nurse can provide an important perspective or make a decision as well as the doctor. Asked whether she wanted to be a leader, Dr. Geordino responded:

> Actually, no. At least, not leadership in the traditional sense. I do see myself as an excellent co-leader. I have no desire to be out front. I don't really care who gets the credit, as long as the right thing is done. I know that's not supposed to be good for women who want to advance in their careers, but I've seen too many people climb over other bodies, trying to

get where they're going. I don't think that's an appropriate way to behave. And that's what I aspire to . . . drive things from beneath. A lot of
things fall through the cracks and no one has the interest or energy to
make sure they happen because there are other issues that are more
pressing. I'm one of those people who will say "This needs to be done,"
and I'll figure out how to get it done.

Dr. Geordino was not interested in self-promotion and getting credit for
her work or even being recognized as a leader. She focused on what
needed to be done, persistence, and ethical standards.

These comments are representative of the attitudes of most women
faculty we spoke to. The use of power described by these leaders is based
on caring and relationship and on creating change that helps people.
They were more oriented toward transparency and were less hierarchical.
Their communal orientation put these female leaders at a disadvantage in
a medical school culture based on individualism and sometimes self-
aggrandizement. Yet, these values also put women in an ideal position to
exercise good leadership, as we will see.

Dr. Westenfelder, who had a great deal of administrative experience,
commented:

I tend to think of power not in the dominance model but in the capacity
model, the ability to get things done. I learned when I was the head of
another organization how seductive power can be. And there are so
many perks and so many ways that people try to curry your favor it can
be distracting and even misleading, and you have to be vigilant all the
time if you want to avoid being seduced by power.

Dr. Haitham's response to a younger colleague's concern over balancing her work life with caring for her toddler demonstrates a commitment
to empowering subordinates:

I spend a lot more time talking to people about their careers and goals to
make sure we're all aligned, that we're moving in the right direction. I had
a conversation with one of my postdocs the other day, a young woman. I
asked her, "How is it going? What do you want to do?" She said, "I'm a
little frustrated because I can't work 'til midnight anymore because I have a

two-year-old child." I said, "Why are you frustrated; don't you enjoy that?" She said, "I do, except that I also want to work." Then she asked me—and I think this was what was bothering her—"Aren't you sorry you hired me; wouldn't you rather have hired someone single?" That's probably what bothers most young women. I said to her, "Absolutely not! In fact I'm extremely happy that I hired you, and I'd be even happier if you could be successful with your family life." That did make a big difference to her.

As a leader, Dr. Francesco also prioritized relationships. Her professional development programs for faculty were geared to creating relationships and trust among them.

> I wanted to make a positive impact; I wanted to help make good things happen for myself and for others. Those were aspirations, and as I moved into positions where I had so-called power or authority or a leadership role or whatever you want to call it, then I would try to create an administrative structure, or a learning environment, that would support those pieces, that would allow things to happen, as opposed to placing barriers in the way of communication, and of the involvement of people in what they're doing. We called it "humanizing the learning environment"
>
> Regarding some of the programs I developed and put in place for the faculty, I was absolutely purposeful in thinking through how I would create this environment, this structure, and those relationships—not just with me, although I was part of it—but between groups of people. So that they could do their learning around whatever it was they were supposed to be learning about. We did it for a number of different content areas. We did it for career-advancement issues, we did it for teaching skills, for writing skills, and cross-cultural communication issues. Then one would hear from the faculty in these collaborative intimate groups that developed how important this environment was for them and how rare it was. The faculty would get to a point where they were able to see that this is transformative. And they would get to the point, as I had felt myself that this was something they had to strive for. They really wanted this. This really helped them in their work, in their relationships, in their teaching.
>
> It's just really rewarding to hear people talk about the effect on themselves. We did a lot of formal evaluation of these programs. We asked them to write about their experience, in very open-ended ways, and so they wrote a lot. They wrote much more about those aspects of the pro-

grams than about the content of the programs. What was most compelling to them, what was of the most value to them, was that they had managed to find themselves within these relationships. I was just blown away by what they said. How wonderful that we managed to do that. Hopefully it will be of some lasting value. And I think, that having given them that experience, they took it back into their work and their teaching.

Initially, the administrative leadership had not really understood Dr. Francesco's change efforts. Eventually, however, when it became apparent that the programs improved faculty morale and skills and the likelihood that they would remain at the school, she gained administrative support.

Dr. Francesco: They tacitly supported it, they allowed it to happen, and gave enough support for it to happen. It became so much part of the fabric of the school and the faculty, that it would have been impossible for them to stop it. At which point they perceived the benefits. In fact, at one point there was some change among the higher ups, and the new school leadership very clearly saw the benefits, and thought it was great.

Dr. Francesco took great personal satisfaction in having created this change by developing an environment that nurtured these trusting relationships. She described that whatever power she had was founded on such relationships.

I had no real authority or power in [the institution], except the power of these relationships. But we did have tremendously successful outcomes. They were recognized internally and then were recognized nationally, too. We wrote about our work, and presented our work, and once we got national recognition, which was of great value to the school (the leadership of the school really liked that piece), that success became associated with me. I never really felt I had any power there, come to think of it. I was on pretty firm ground though, and I didn't feel that vulnerable in the work I was doing anymore, despite not having real power. It was just the power of these relationships.

Dr. Westenfelder, as an experienced administrator, clearly articulated her conceptual framework for effective leadership. She linked authority to values and to acting in ways that earned trust and respect.

Dr. Westenfelder: One of the biggest challenges in leadership, whatever level you're at, whether it's positional leadership or whether it's informal leadership, is balancing justice and compassion. Looking out for the good of the group versus looking out for the good of the individual. Trying to serve both of those eventually requires you to be courageous. Because if you serve justice there will be some people who don't want justice, who really don't want the balance, and will come after you. It'll be unpopular. And in the instances where you serve compassion, there are also some people sometimes who don't really want some people to have compassion. Being a good leader means that you should always be acting in a way that deserves other people's trust and respect, but it also means that not everybody is going to like you or what you do. You need to be strong enough to do something because it's the best thing.

Dr. Westenfelder is in fact describing the transformational style of leadership defined by Burns, which is characterized by trust (see Chapter 4). The benefits of trusting leaders have been studied extensively, and trust is a key concept in several theoretical frameworks for effective leadership. Burns makes a distinction between leaders who are "power wielders" and those who fit his framework of moral leadership. In his view, the values of leaders and followers must be aligned in order for trust to develop and for the leaders to be effective. Burns specifically says, "We must see power—and leadership—as not things but as relationships," adding that relationship failures and lack of trust prevent a leader from being effective for very long (Burns 1978).

The transformational approach to leadership, exemplified by Drs. Westenfelder and Francesco, turns out to be more common among women, as a large body of research indicates. A meta-analysis of over 160 studies showed that women's style of leadership is more participative or democratic (communal) and less autocratic or directive (agentic) than men's (Eagly and Johnson 1990). Other studies concluded that men are more self-assertive and dominant and show less deference and warmth toward team members than women (Carli and Eagly 1999) and that female managers are more likely to adopt a more transformational style of leadership (Eagly et al. 2003). Women managers and executives consistently score higher on behavioral skills such as team work, empowerment, sharing information, and care for employees. The research indicates that this difference between women and men tends to be smaller in highly male-dominated settings such as academic medicine. In our interviews, women wanted to empower the people they led and worked to create groups based on relationship and trust. Those who were fortunate enough to have been mentored noted that the mentors who took time to nurture and support them were women. No doubt some women do have male mentors (as I have had myself), but our sample of interviewees did not describe such an experience.

Another quality that emerges from our interviews, which is extremely important for effective leadership, is what Goleman termed "emotional intelligence," the awareness of one's own and other people's emotions (Goleman 1998). Goleman says that women tend to be more aware of their emotions, show more empathy, and are more adept interpersonally than men. Other studies have demonstrated that women physicians communicate more effectively with patients (Roter and Hall 1992). This quality of emotional intelligence contributes to the reasons why women are the ones who often wind up looking after the students; they perceive and are able to respond to the students' emotional needs. We have also seen Drs. Booker, Haitham, and Goldsmith all talking about feelings as a significant component of their leadership. Dr. Francesco, also, felt that whatever power she exerted within her institution arose largely from the relationships she had built. Dr. Haitham was careful to support her postdoctoral student with a young child; and as we will see, she believed that an important effect of leadership was to make her a more empathic person herself.

How Leadership Changed Women

Women leaders not only changed their institutions; they discovered that assuming leadership led to changes in themselves. Their character and abilities evolved; so did their capacity to help and nurture others and their feelings about their institution. Many interviewees said or implied that the institutional recognition they received as leaders played an important part in giving them a sense of really belonging. For instance, Dr. Rose didn't see herself as a member of the university or the medical school community "until I was put in a position where I had to try to lead a subset of that community."

Dr. Brown, an Emergency Medicine physician, said that the Dean's recognition of her competence to take over a leadership position in the university was critical:

> When I first came, he said, I don't know if you can do this job. I said, "Okay, fair enough." And then, about eight months later, he tells me, "It's clear you can do the job. I want you to be part of a small group of people who help move this institution forward." And it has really been rewarding for me to have him say that. It's made me even more feel a commitment to the institution.

Dr. Rouge also responded positively to being included in decision making:

> I've had my first serious experience of power and leadership in the past year and a half as the vice-chair and then the chair of an important committee. I have to admit it's heady, it's an awful lot of fun, it's nice to have your opinion respected, it's great to be part of things and included in decisions and to actually be able to set priorities and have people say to you, "What do you think?" and have that matter. It has not really been part of my experience before now. I had to get to this age to get a taste of that.

Dr. Haitham felt that being in a leadership role helped her become more self-confident and more empowering and supportive of the people she supervised.

> It certainly has given me confidence, and then in terms of relationships it affected me in two ways: one, in my relationship to the people who may be my peers or who are above me in the stratification or social hierarchy, and two, with people who report to me, who are below me in the hierarchy. The thing that bothered me about integrity and ethics—I have felt empowered to speak out as much as I can and need to in public about these issues. That has made me feel self-confident and secure in terms of people above me. Regarding the people below me, it has affected me in the sense of becoming a little more sensitive.
>
> I was a workaholic in the sense that I worked very hard because I always felt that to succeed or not be embarrassed, I had to do better than

everyone around me. But it's interesting that I don't expect this from others in my group. Even now [laugh] I may be the hardest working, actually. And I have a lot of empathy for them. So I think that self-confidence has made me much more empathetic to people who have other sides of their lives, than perhaps when I wasn't successful and powerful. Because then, I was anxious when the people weren't working and things weren't getting done and I was thinking "there goes the grant" and all of that.

Leadership and power really provided a possibility for me to be, if you will, in the old jargon, a kinder human being, which is ultimately what life's about. So I think that's really helped a lot, and I'm grateful to have been relatively successful.

The self-confidence Dr. Haitham derived from her position allowed her to speak out about ethical issues to her peers and supervisors and also to be more sensitive and empathetic to her junior colleagues. Dr. Haitham actually grew into the person she wanted to be as she learned how to exercise a form of power that suited her character and beliefs. She said, "I think that's the best part of getting these positions, a benefit of leadership."

Looking at these women in the light of the "tempered radical" concept, it seems that although they felt marginal, they were able to turn that difference into a positive attribute and use it to create change. Rhoda Unger, a noted gender psychologist, suggests that women's sense of marginality may help them feel more comfortable occupying a position "in the big leagues," since it allows them not to take responsibility for all the negative attributes they perceive in leaders and which they want to avoid themselves. This freedom from feeling responsible for what is wrong with the system may help women be more effective leaders and enable them to address inequities such as disparities in health care and dehumanizing aspects of the patient's experience.

Why Some Leave Leadership

Dr. Tonder: I wasn't able to get beyond the department to the level of the medical school and the institution to affect the kind of change that I thought needed to happen. And that's when I really became disappointed, and I felt I was no longer being successful about things that were important that I should have been able to achieve at that level.

Like Dr. Tonder, a number of women leaders stayed only a short time in their positions; they left because they were not willing to compromise their values to conform to the status quo in their medical schools. These women continued to feel like outsiders even though they had been extremely successful and accomplished—and were so again once they left the organization in question. Some were so wounded emotionally and professionally that they left academic medicine completely and entered new highly successful careers in higher education institutions.

One such leader, Dr. Frank, left after coming up against an intransigent superior in her medical school's administration who, rather than take advantage of her potential contributions, felt it safer to remove her from the school.

> Dr. Frank: What excited me about the [leadership] position was that I thought I would finally have the authority to put in place new structures or programs, or a way of operating, and I felt that this work would be supported. Not that I could do it all myself, but the barriers at the top would be removed to having this sort of change-work done, because I had such a high position (I thought I had such a position; inherent in [my] title was that authority). Additionally, it was my impression from the interview process of meeting with many faculty and students, but particularly faculty—maybe 40 interviews—that they really wanted this change to happen. They didn't know what they wanted, but they really wanted change. And so I thought, this is just a most exciting opportunity, to walk into it and set up a way of helping this change happen . . . you'd think, "Wow!!! We could really make a change here, really affect the culture" and make it so that this really filters down to the students and the way they learn and to the whole education process.
>
> However, there was a lot about the position I didn't know and that was kept from me—quite purposefully. So when in this new role I started to move in those directions, the faculty were very supportive and excited to be participating, and we started to take steps to make this sort of thing happen. They started to talk about how this was different from anything else that had happened there. And then they started to warn me about the leadership in the school; it was only really one person, to whom I reported, but they kept warning me. I thought "No, it will be all right, everybody wants this to happen here."

But eventually I came to understand that the long-standing top leader did not want this to happen and perceived it to be extremely threatening. He totally undermined the whole thing because he had ultimate power and chose to use it. The last thing he wanted was transparency and intimacy and empowerment of people and real change, because it threatened his own position so greatly, threatened his control.

My response to being undermined was just to work harder to make it happen because the faculty so wanted it to succeed. Faculty *and* the students—everybody was really cheering on this whole process. My thinking was, "If the leadership really sees what good stuff will come out of this, that it will benefit them as well as everyone else, they can take part credit for it, then it'll work." But it was naïve of me to think that. The writing was on the wall right from the beginning. I was used as a sort of sop to the faculty; the faculty wanted change, so let them choose someone who they think can bring in change. I can only assume that the long-standing leadership felt that I would be prepared to go along with business as usual. But I wasn't, and that was my problem.

They recognized very early on that I was in effect incorruptible. That was why I was so dangerous. They couldn't make me go along with the way they conducted business. Then, they had to figure out some way of getting me out of that place. In the beginning, faculty were totally supportive and would send me e-mails saying "Thank God you bring a different set of values to this place, but you do realize you're in real dangerous territory here," and a lot of people individually came to warn me. But it was only in retrospect I realized what they were all saying. Those same faculty who had been so supportive and so wanted this change to work—when it became apparent to them that "the leaders" were dead against it, they retreated into a culture of silence because they were all so fearful for their own positions. They were all frightened of being seen to be aligned with me, who was "somebody" no longer—persona non grata. They felt so vulnerable that the only way they could behave was to compromise their own values and what they wanted.

This individual is one example of a number of women leaders whose unwillingness to compromise their values was apparently one factor contributing to their limited staying power in positions of authority. These leaders left their positions relatively soon after taking them, seeking a different working environment. While in office, they felt scrutinized and evaluated rather than supported and treated with some generosity of spirit. And then, usually fairly suddenly and without explanation, they no longer had their positions. Some lingered on—as professors or in some other job—until they found a new position, or they just disappeared. In their own institutions, there was generally little public discourse as to why, but rather a muffled undercurrent of rumor and conjecture.

We have seen that, contrary to widespread assumptions, women medical faculty are ambitious and do want to be leaders—being wives and mothers does not stop them—but that they face both internal and external barriers to achieving positions of power and authority. Those who do make it into leadership are frequently prevented from achieving their full potential by institutional resistance to change. Yet, as this chapter has explained, women could bring to the medical school an empowering, democratic, transformative type of leadership that has been shown to be effective in other sectors and I believe would bring many benefits to academic medicine. These intelligent, courageous, energetic women leaders should be allowed to make their full contributions to their fields and to the nation.

REFERENCES

Burns JM. Leadership. New York: Harper & Row; 1978.

Carli LL, Eagly AH. Gender effects on influence and emergent leadership. In: Powell GN, ed. Handbook of gender and work. Thousand Oaks, CA: Sage; 1999:203–22.

Catalyst. Census of women corporate officers and top earners. New York: Catalyst; 2000.

Eagly AH, Johannesen-Schmidt MC, van Engen M, Vinkenburg C. Transformational, transactional, and laissez-faire leadership styles: A meta-analysis comparing women and men. Psychol Bull. 2003;129(4):569–91.

Eagly AH, Johnson BT. Gender and leadership style: a meta-analysis. Psychol Bull. 1990;108:233–56.

Eagly AH, Karau SJ. Role congruity theory of prejudice toward female leaders. Psychol Rev. 2002;109:573–98.

Eagly AH, Makhijani MG, Klonsky BG. Gender and the evaluation of leaders: a meta-analysis. Psychol Bull. 1992;111:3–22.

Fels A. Do women lack ambition? Harvard Bus Rev. 2004;82(4):50–60.

Flower J. Leadership without easy answers. A conversation with Ronald Heifetz. Healthcare Forum 1995. Available at http://www.well.com/~bbear/heifetz.html.

Goleman D. Working with emotional intelligence. New York: Bantam; 1998.

Heifetz RA, Linsky M. Leadership on the line. Boston: Harvard Business School Press; 2002.

Heilman ME. Description and prescription: how gender stereotypes prevent women's ascent up the organizational ladder. J Social Issues. 2001;57:657–74.

Kanter RM. Men and women of the corporation. New York: Basic Books; 1977.

Palmer PJ. Let your life speak: listening for the voice of vocation. San Francisco: Jossey-Bass; 1999.

Roter DL, Hall JL. Doctors talking with patients/patients talking with doctors: improving communication in medical visits. Westport, CT: Auburn House; 1992.

Schein V. A global look at psychological barriers to women's progress in management. J Social Issues. 2001;57:675–88.

Chapter 8   Developing a Critical Consciousness for Change

{ New leadership is needed for new times, but it will not come from finding more wily ways to manipulate the external world. It will come as we who serve and teach and lead find the courage to take an inner journey toward both our shadows and our light—a journey that, faithfully pursued, will take us beyond ourselves to become healers of a wounded world. —Parker J. Palmer (2009) }

What are the responsibilities of academic medicine to society, to health care, and to patients? Traditionally, its mission has been tripartite: research, education, and patient care. Yet the preceding chapters have painted a portrait of institutions that frequently undervalue their teaching mission, fail to fully recognize and reward excellence in patient care (when not expensive or high-tech), and are inattentive to social justice issues, such as ensuring health care access and equal medical services for all people. These institutions demand relentless work, yet devote scant effort to adequately supporting the human needs of their faculty members who serve as physicians, teachers, and scientists. They reward individualism rather than collaboration and at times overlook ethical lapses.

Faculty may feel conflicted when they perceive their institution to be out of sync with their own basic personal and professional values. They see a decline in humanism in medicine. Faculty find that their experience of work and the values exhibited by their organizations fail to honor their "heart," and for this reason they often do not do their best work; finding their work less meaningful, they become morally distressed and emotionally exhausted. Many eventually leave academic medicine. Leaders, too, feel lonely and vulnerable, as well as besieged by fiscal responsibilities.

The goal of this book is not, however, to leave readers with a despairing picture of academic medicine. Its many and real successes are described daily in the mass media and scholarly journals. The goal is rather to point out that the medical faculty as it currently exists actually constitutes a highly idealistic, competent, and compassionate group—a vital resource with the potential not only to transform the culture of the medical school but also to be at the forefront of changing our entire system of health care for the better.

This book has focused on interview data from women, but men we interviewed for our studies described comparable feelings of invisibility and isolation and the same negative effects of the culture of individualism as the women quoted in Chapter 4. Men also often felt a similar distress about lack of alignment between their values and those they saw in their institution. The reason I focused the book on women is that, precisely because of their outsider status, their perceptions of the medical school's organizational approach serve as a window into this sometimes unhealthy culture, enabling us to see it more clearly—the first step toward change.

Because of their marginalization, minority and nonminority women (and underrepresented minority male faculty as well) are more able to see the bias and exclusion that may operate in academic medical centers, as well as other problematic dimensions of the culture. In our work on cultural identity, we found that when different groups of people are asked to describe their own culture, the group least readily able to do so is the dominant majority. This book, therefore, has looked closely at women's experiences in academic medicine in order to shine a light on that culture as a whole. A next step is to use their awareness (and that of minority groups) to develop a broader vision of what that culture should be and can be like. This is one reason why we urgently need more diversity in medical school leadership. Women and people of color can drive crucial changes in education, research, and patient care, because their own experience shows them clearly how current practices are not meeting the needs of faculty, students, patients, and the population as a whole. Providing this critical consciousness and clarity of vision, followed by action for change, is the potential gift of these groups.

Four basic issues must be addressed:

- The moral integrity and professional tenets of medical care are compromised.
- The system does not take full account of patients, physicians and scientists as human beings.

- Medical school students—the next generation of physicians—are not receiving the education, emotional support, and role modeling they require to develop their professional values and commitments, and identity as physicians.
- The present culture of academic medicine is causing substantial distress among many of its own faculty, preventing them from making the full contributions they are capable of.

A Morally Compromised System

Large numbers of idealistic women and men choose to enter the profession of medicine, but the present ethos of academic medical centers often becomes a barrier to putting their ideals into practice. As indicated in our interviews, the culture frequently fails to support the values that contributed to the choice of a career in medicine. The organizational culture does support intellectual rigor, but not so much the social mission.

The much talked about crisis in health care is evidence of the inadequacy of our health care system. We spend more than any other country on health care, but rank last among 19 industrialized nations on health outcomes, quality, and efficiency, according to a report by the Commonwealth Foundation. Over 46 million people lack access to medical care because they don't have health "insurance," and millions more receive inadequate care. We also have serious disparities in health care and outcomes among certain sectors of the population, often related to race and poverty. These disparities are a glaring national problem, in addition to that of the number of people with no access to medical services. (Sweeping health care reform legislation of March 2010 has somewhat addressed economic inequality and access, even though it has not unchained health care from the private insurance industry.)

Such an unequal health care system is not ethical, and the physicians who work in academic medicine are aware of this. Failure to live up to the professional tenet of social justice and providing health care to all, with equal access and equal care—regardless of social circumstances, ability to pay, race or ethnicity—results in many faculty feeling morally compromised. Women, particularly, are often disheartened by the lack of congruence between their own professional values and those acted out and supported by their medical school organizations. The professional principles of truthfulness and always prioritizing the patient's well being over personal or institutional gain are also sometimes compromised by power and privilege, the medical industrial complex, medical insurance companies, and pharmaceutical companies.

There is a parallel between the lack of diversity—whether of gender or of race—in academic medicine and the different levels of service that our health care system provides to different groups. Lack of diversity is also a reason for our health care system's falling short of excellence. Without including diverse perspectives, it is improbable to create an optimal health care system for our multicultural population. Diversity drives excellence.

Relationships and the Human Side of Faculty

This book has addressed the human needs of medical professionals. Both women and men faculty cherish positive relationships with their patients and students but often feel isolated and disconnected from colleagues and leaders. Many say that humanistic qualities are undervalued in the highly competitive institutional reward system that fosters individualistic, rather than collaborative behavior. Many medical faculty feel excluded and disrespected; they develop few good relationships and distrust many colleagues and leaders. As we saw, medical faculty cannot bring their whole selves to their workplace and thus are unable to do their best work.

This lack of healthy human connections in academic medicine leads to another undesirable parallel: dehumanized faculty will tend to treat patients and medical students the same way they themselves are treated. The decline in humanism in medicine contributes to poor communication between doctors and patients, patients who are dissatisfied with their care and are less likely to follow medical advice, and distrust in the medical system among the population at large. It seems likely that this disconnectedness contributes to unprofessional behavior and attrition.

Devaluing of Medical Education

Medical schools are the only venue to educate physicians. Research can be conducted elsewhere, but only a medical school can grant an MD degree. This is why the teaching mission of the medical school is critical to our national health care system, and it is thus ironic that of all medical school activities, education is least valued. Many faculty feel passionate about innovation and the quality of medical education; they see it as the opportunity to mold the next generation of physicians. Unfortunately, medical schools do not prioritize this part of their mission, and faculty who devote time and intellectual effort to teaching are not adequately recognized and supported. In addition, given what we have seen of stress and moral distress among medical school faculty, it is not surprising that medical students do not always develop into kind, compassionate physicians but instead become less altruistic and more cynical during their medical school years.

Faculty Distress

Academic medical center faculty are a vanguard: critical in providing sophisticated clinical care, creating new knowledge through research, and teaching the nation's next generation of doctors. They are the most precious resource in academic medicine; they drive and influence every aspect of care, research, and education. The vitality and attitudes of faculty in turn influence the lessons learned by medical students. There is little hope for changing the culture if we do not help the faculty become more energized and inspired, since creating change requires that they function optimally. Yet they are leaving academic medicine at an alarming rate. We need to help faculty move beyond the professional expectations of their formal titles and bring more of their whole person to the conversation. Faculty need guidance in developing self-awareness and time to reflect on the meaningfulness of their work.

The Complexity of Change

An institutional culture and learning environment that supports altruism and excellence, welcomes diversity, encourages innovation, is characterized by trust, and models the positive qualities we need in physicians is absolutely essential. Nonetheless, an academic medical center is a highly complex institution and bringing change to it is an equally complex undertaking. The culture is very resistant to change. People seek quick fixes, but in such a system, change cannot happen quickly or easily. The information presented in this book is an attempt to enhance awareness of needs and point to possibilities. One important element of culture change is actually understanding the current culture, and our interviews and this book are such an exploration. The following sections lay out major areas in which changes could bring about a shift in medical school culture.

Creating Relationship

The basic message of this book is a call for a core change in medical school culture that encourages connections and trusting relationships among colleagues and supports the human needs of health professionals. We are all profoundly affected by the social context in which we work. Medical schools need to build social structures and learning environments for all their sectors—students, residents, faculty, administration, and staff—that are mutually respectful, nurturing, and compassionate. People are the lifeblood of the organization. An organization functions as a network of conversations, communications, and relationships; it is largely the collective ideas of its members. Every meeting is an opportunity to make relationships. Introducing purposeful relational practices has led to substantial increases in productivity in the business sector, and our own data suggest that behaviors promoting relationship formation can mitigate stress and may help prevent burnout (Catalyst n.d.; Deloitte 2003). Creating better interpersonal connections across the systems of health care would improve communication and collaborative efforts in patient care, research, education, and administration, and lead to a faculty with more vocational vitality and satisfaction.

Academic medicine leaders need to learn to trust in and be compassionate with faculty, recognizing their motivations and best qualities. Previous chapters have already described cases where establishing trust and good relationships yielded very positive outcomes: Dr. Francesco's creation of faculty professional development programs that created humanistic environments and relationships among faculty members; Dr. Mere, the department chair, who described being a mother as an advantage when caring for her faculty members; the changes made by Dr. Goldsmith in her surgery department and by Dr. Haitham in her research laboratory.

Longtime colleagues Drs. Thomas Inui, Rich Frankel, Debra Litzelman, Penny Williamson, and Tony Suchman initiated a school-wide culture change project using a participatory approach at Indiana University School of Medicine. They gathered and presented stories of the school's culture "at its best" to foster mindfulness of positive relational patterns already present in the environment. Their work prompted significant un-anticipated shifts in ordinary activities and behavior, including a rede-signed admissions process for medical students, new relational practices at faculty meetings, and modifications of administrative practices such as departmental performance reviews (Cottingham et al. 2008).

Consciously Welcoming and Working to Achieve Diversity

As we saw, women and people of color feel marginalized and invisible; they are often discriminated against and excluded from decision making and from powerful positions. Yet the system needs their perspectives in leadership positions. We cannot address the problems of health care op-timally unless we include all these additional voices, and we can only fully accomplish that if we change the culture so that they are welcomed and valued, and their different perspectives recognized and honored. In-stitutional leaders need to welcome—or, preferably, seek out—and listen to diverse opinions from outsider groups. Diverse voices generate a richer situational analysis by contributing new insights to planning and decision making around complex issues.

I believe that achieving diversity represents the greatest opportunity for addressing more effectively the nation's current health care needs, and also for enhancing collaborative research. As we heard from our inter-viewees, a rich potential for change already exists in the hearts and minds of women and underrepresented minority faculty acting as "tempered radicals," some of whom are already creating positive changes.

It would also be extremely valuable for current leaders to explore their own values, assumptions, and biases. Majority men of good conscience need to use their power to mandate the inclusion of women and both male and female people of color at the highest echelons of academic med-icine. Supporting the values and ideals of these groups as they move into leadership positions will reorient the culture. As tempered radicals, they not only enrich our perspectives and capabilities in academic medicine, but also serve as powerful role models for the next generation. As Dr. Goldsmith put it:

> If you had a more flexible system that allowed more of the gadflies and
> oddballs to get through, you'd end up with these different thinking

people. I do think you'd have solutions that were better and you would be better off because of that.

Even though the care of women and vulnerable populations is a responsibility of all physicians, we know that women and underrepresented minority faculty are more likely to champion research about women's health and health disparities and to serve underserved communities; these groups must be encouraged to lead in addressing these goals for the nation.

Changing the Culture

A century ago, a seminal report by educator Abraham Flexner led to wide-ranging reforms of medical education in the United States. Today, the uncontrollable and unsustainable cost of U.S. health care and its unjust distribution make it imperative that our medical schools empower a wider range of professionals to provide inspirational and effective leadership. Doing so will require a fundamental change in the culture of medical schools and teaching hospitals, which shape American health care.

The professional ideals of academic medicine call on it to lead the way in reforming health care. Medical leaders need to support the values and professional ideals of their faculty so that the faculty's passion for improving medical practice begins to drive more of the core activities of medical schools—thus influencing the next generation of researchers and physicians in training. The values and priorities of any organization are implicit in how it organizes and structures its administration and work. Having shared values among leaders and faculty would increase the leaders' effectiveness and enable them to be "transformational." We must reverse the current trend, which gives development and funding of new knowledge in the biomedical and clinical sciences, along with pressure to increase clinical "productivity," priority over social activism, medical education, a reflective process on values, the personal needs of faculty, and professional development.

As we heard in our interviews, women in leadership roles feel strongly that the present system has to change. As women, they feel atypical within the existing structures and may hold differing values. Women think that the system can be successful only if it changes to accommodate and reflect differences from traditional and paternalistic methods and attitudes.

Drs. Goldsmith and Westenfelder are examples of tempered radicals who have managed to resist the imposition of current organizational mores. Significantly, they both suggested that the new generation of faculty, men as well as women, would not tolerate the current system. As Dr. Westenfelder put it:

> I really believe that in a lot of medical schools right now, the faculty are pretty close to the red zone, both men and women. . . . And I think it'll be the Generation X men who provide the energy to finally have it change, because they are not going to tolerate it either—they aren't tolerating it already. It's going to take a generation, at least, to restructure, because it isn't just about restructuring academic medicine; it's embedded in the health care system.

Men and women both are seeking more flexibility in their work life and a better balance between their personal and professional responsibilities. Not addressing this need will cause further attrition from academic medicine.

Another aspect of the culture that must change is its attitude to education. Promoting the teaching mission of a medical school and recognizing it as a center of excellence in medical education requires a guiding administrative structure that enhances the prestige of teaching, rewards outstanding teachers, and nurtures junior faculty. Providing faculty with resources; recognizing teaching; educational innovation and scholarship; and assisting faculty with programs addressing the learning environment and teaching skills will help ensure the faculty's vitality and academic productivity and keep them in their jobs.

In addition, medical students must be guided in a reflective process about their roles as physicians and how this role is related to social justice and the real privilege of being a physician. Along with the faculty, students must take an inward journey to examine their own values and beliefs in order to respond with integrity to the competing demands of their chosen vocation (Palmer 1999).

To create this culture change, we need leaders who have insight into the present culture, are aware of their own values and biases, and have acquired some cultural humility and objectivity. We can't change a top-down model by using hierarchical approaches. Such an assumption aligns with Heifitz' concept of creating a structure within which to engage the hearts and minds of organizational members. Leaders are facilitators and supporters rather than experts who know the answers. This environment would draw on the energy of the numberless conversations taking place in an organization and use them to bring about culture change (Brown and Isaacs 2005). It seems that successful organizational change is determined by the participation of many people and is a more emergent and adaptive process.

Traditionally trained and reinforced leaders from within the organization may be unwilling and unable to contemplate and drive such change. Transformative and effective leaders may need to come in increasing numbers from outsiders—women and people of color. In the words of Edgar Schein, a nationally recognized expert on organizational psychology at MIT, "the leader must be a skilled change manager who first learns what the present state of the culture is, unfreezes it, redefines and changes it" (Schein 1992).

The C - Change Experiment

Culture change happens very slowly, but even early in the action phase of the C - Change Initiative, developments with the potential to introduce real change had become apparent. Our Learning Action Network process (see p. 8) embodied a type of culture change where we attempted to connect the intellect with emotion and engage in a collaborative and noncompetitive manner. It was Diversity in Action. The C - Change deans were willing to have their faculty confidentially interviewed, and they listened to diverse points of view. As Learning Action Network members, the dean and faculty studied the findings from our interviews and then confronted the information we heard; learned about the social science literature on nonconscious bias and marginalization (see chapter 6); and incorporated learning about organizational psychology and change from outside medicine. The group entered into dialogue about the meaning of this work, its relevance to their own institutional goals, contexts, and resources and to the part that they as individuals played in their various positions.

Drawing on the principles and practices of the Center for Courage and Renewal, we encouraged the deans and faculty to reflect, using journaling, poetry, and dialogue to facilitate examining their own values and beliefs and how these related to the competing demands of their roles and responsibilities. We tried to get to the heart of the matter. Concurrently, a basic belief we hold is that human systems grow toward what they persistently ask questions about. Using this concept early in the process, the group came up with a set of so-called "Evergreen Questions." We hoped that these would be enduring questions that would serve as guides for decision making and planning for complex change. These questions could help us to be sure that the work we were doing would result in the changes and accomplishments that we sought. Examples were: How will this support the growth and learning of all involved? How will this support relationship formation? Is this appreciative of the faculty? How would this make our faculty feel supported and respected? Would this help our faculty identify and reach their goals and aspirations? How will this promote and value diversity? Are we engaging relevant stakeholders and keeping them engaged? We often used methods to encourage dialogue and conversations that matter such as World Café (Brown and Isaacs 2005) and Appreciative Inquiry, which focuses attention on what has worked best to drive positive change (Cooperrider et al. 2000).

In response to this work, the different C - Change schools have implemented various changes; some funded new positions—"deans for multiculturalism and diversity"—responsible for examining and addressing inclusion and diversity issues. Some held leadership retreats and educational programs, informed their trustees about the issues raised during these events, and invited opinions from community and underrepresented minority faculty. Based on what they had learned about nonconscious bias, some began educating their faculty search committees about this issue. They considered the goal of inclusion and developed a more sophisticated awareness of diverse views within their faculties. Finally, some began working toward creating new policies and programs. Each of these actions and innovations resulted in some culture change—for what leadership says is important *is* the culture. Even in these times of budgetary constraints, much of this work can continue and is not funding intensive. If a leader shows up for a meeting about diversity, that in itself changes the culture. Making the choice to do something—to take some steps—rather than doing nothing because of the huge complexity—is a stride to long-term and meaningful change. C - Change schools have been brave in considering just such change.

Trust as a Hallmark of Success

A critical component often missing from the current culture is trust. In fact, a high level of trust is a hallmark of a successful health care system. Again we see a parallel relationship between the inside and outside of the academic medical establishment: just as the people within the system don't trust each other, the patients who turn to the system for needed care don't trust it to look after them adequately. We should consider our health care system fully successful only if its members have trust in their relationships with colleagues, students, or teachers, and if the people it serves feel that they can trust the care they receive. To realize the potential of all faculty, including women and people of color, a logical response to the findings of our studies would be to facilitate a core change in medical school culture that encourages and supports connection in trusting relationships and the human condition of health professionals. We need to invoke an educational approach that could help make the connection between the mindset and "heartset" of our faculty and medical school leaders. This would open the way to the full flowering of both women's and men's potential contributions and skills.

The Real Work

It may be that when we no longer know what
to do we have come to our real work
and that when we no longer know which way
to go we have begun our real journey.
The mind that is not baffled is not employed.
The impeded stream is the one that sings.
  — *Wendell Berry, from* Standing by Words: Essays

REFERENCES

Brown J, Isaacs D, World Café Community. The World Café: Shaping our futures through conversations that matter. San Francisco: Berrett-Koehler Pubs; 2005.
Catalyst. Available at http://catalyst.org.
Cooperrider DL, Sorensen PF, Whitney D, Yaeger TF, eds. Appreciative inquiry:

rethinking human organization toward a positive theory of change. Champaign, IL: Stipes Publishing; 2000.

Cottingham AH, Suchman AL, Litzelman DK, Frankel RM, Mossbarger DL, Williamson PR, Baldwin D, Inui T. Enhancing the informal curriculum of a medical school: a case study in organizational culture change. J Gen Intern Med. 2008;23(6):715–22.

Deloitte. 2003. Women's initiative. Available at: http://www.deloitte.com.

Palmer PJ. Let your life speak: listening for the voice of vocation. San Francisco: Jossey-Bass; 1999.

Palmer PJ. 2009. Available at: http://www.couragerenewal.org/newsletter/issue1/54-.

Schein E. Organizational culture and leadership. San Francisco: Jossey-Bass; 1992.

In writing this book, I also wished to provide those in leadership roles in medical schools a window into some unexpected and disturbing experiences of medical faculty that they may not be aware of. I sincerely hope that these leaders do not perceive this book as an overstated or indiscriminate indictment of their complex and in most ways highly successful programs but, instead, gain insights from this book that will facilitate their faculty recruitment and retention, and enhance growth and excellence in their institutions. Additionally, it has been my intent all along to honor intrepid women in medicine. As Lani Guinier said, "We have a gift, not a grievance."

I strongly encourage any bright and idealistic young woman or man to go into medicine. This book was not planned as a deterrent but as an inspiration for physicians in training or those contemplating a life as a doctor. They need to be determined and persistent in building a culture for themselves that will embody and retain the spirit with which they enter the richly rewarding profession of medicine. I offer this book to medical students, physicians and scientists who speak out and stand up for equity, civility, diversity, and patient- and relationship-centered care, in addition to contributing to medical research and teaching.

> If you want to identify me, ask me not where I live, or what I like to eat, or how I comb my hair, but ask me what I am living for, in detail, ask me what I think is keeping me from living fully for the thing I want to live for.
>
> —*Thomas Merton*